C000151604

This volume describes a complementary selection of tests to those described in the companion volume *Basic Mutagenicity Tests* (Cambridge, 1990). These supplementary tests are used to assess risks of *in vitro* mutagenicity in those instances where the basic tests are inconclusive. As such, these tests have an important role in the assessment of the safety of new compounds, drugs and chemicals.

These supplementary tests and guidelines, originally drawn up by the United Kingdom Environmental Mutagen Society (UKEMS) several years ago, have now been fully revised and updated in this publication to take full account of new regulatory guidelines and scientific advances.

This volume is therefore an essential source of reference and practical guidance for everyone involved in regulatory affairs, mutagenicity testing, and the successful registration of new chemical products in the UK and the rest of Europe.

There are two companion volumes to this publication:

Basic Mutagenicity Tests: UKEMS Recommended Procedures D. J. KIRKLAND
An essential guide to the four main test procedures for measuring mutagenicity: bacterial mutation assays, metaphase chromosome aberration assays *in vitro*, gene mutation assays in cultured mammalian cells and *in vivo* cytogenetic assays.

Statistical Evaluation of Mutagenicity Test Data D. J. KIRKLAND
This companion UKEMS volume provides a rigorous and practical account of the design and statistical interpretation of mutagenicity tests.

Other titles of interest:

A Practical Approach to Toxicological Investigations A. POOLE & B. LESLIE
This is a useful introduction to toxicology, largely in the context of testing new drugs. It addresses issues such as the selection and performance of suitable toxicological studies.

In-vitro *Methods in Toxicology* C. K. ATTERWILL & C. E. STEELE
This book describes the use of tissue-culture techniques to screen for drug-induced toxicity. It will be of great practical value to all professional toxicologists who are making use of these increasingly important techniques.

Calculated Risks: The Toxicity and Human Health Hazards of Chemicals in our Environment J. RODRICKS
A clear-sighted account of the dangers, real and imagined, from the widespread use of chemicals in our environment.

Supplementary mutagenicity tests

Supplementary mutagenicity tests: UKEMS recommended procedures

UKEMS sub-committee on guidelines for mutagenicity testing. Report. Part II revised

EDITORS
David J. Kirkland
Margaret Fox

ASSOCIATE EDITORS
Terry M. Brooks
James C. Kennelly
Carl N. Martin
Charles Tease
L. Michael Holmstrom

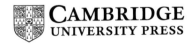 CAMBRIDGE
UNIVERSITY PRESS

Published by the Press Syndicate of the University of Cambridge
The Pitt Building, Trumpington Street, Cambridge CB2 1RP
40 West 20th Street, New York, NY 10011–4211, USA
10 Stamford Road, Oakleigh, Melbourne 3166, Australia

© United Kingdom Environmental Mutagen Society 1993

First published 1993

Printed in Great Britain at the University Press, Cambridge

A catalogue record for this book is available from the British Library

Library of Congress cataloguing in publication data

Supplementary mutagenicity tests: UKEMS recommended procedures:
report, part II revised / UKEMS Subcommittee on Guidelines for
Mutagenicity Testing; editors, David J. Kirkland, Margaret Fox;
associate editors, Terry M. Brooks . . . [et al.]
    p. cm.
Companion volume to Basic mutagenicity tests.
Includes bibliographical references and index.
ISBN 0-521-45073-X
1. Mutagenicity testing. I. Kirkland, David J. II. Fox,
Margaret. III. Brooks, Terry M. IV. United Kingdom Environmental
Mutagen Society. Sub-Committee on Guidelines for Mutagenicity
Testing. V. Basic mutagenicity tests.
QH465.A1U55 1990 Suppl.
616'.042–dc 20   93–17307 CIP

ISBN 0 521 45073 X hardback

WD

CONTENTS

STEERING GROUP

Margaret Fox, Paterson Institute for Cancer Research, Christie Hospital and Holt Radium Institute, Manchester M20 9BX, UK

David J. Kirkland, Hazleton Microtest, Otley Road, Harrogate, North Yorkshire HG3 1PY, UK

John Ashby, Zeneca plc, Central Toxicology Laboratory, Alderley Park, Macclesfield, Cheshire SK10 4TJ, UK

Bryn A. Bridges, MRC Cell Mutation Unit, Sussex University, Falmer, Brighton BN1 9RR, UK

Robert D. Combes, School of Maths and Sciences, LSU College of Higher Education, The Avenue, Southampton, Hants SO9 5HB, UK

Robin J. Fielder, Department of Health, Hannibal House, Elephant and Castle, London SE1 6TE, UK

David G. Gatehouse, Genetic and Reproductive Toxicology Department, Glaxo Group Research Ltd, Ware, Hertfordshire SG12 0DJ, UK

Patricia P. Koundakjian, Health and Safety Executive, Magdalen House, Stanley Precinct, Bootle, Merseyside L20 3QZ, UK

James M. Parry, Molecular Biology Research Group, University College of Swansea, Singleton Park, Swansea SA2 8PP, UK

CONTRIBUTORS

John Ashby, Zeneca plc, Central Toxicology Laboratory, Alderley Park, Macclesfield, Cheshire SK10 4TJ, UK

Diane J. Benford, Robens Institute of Health and Safety, University of Surrey, Guildford, Surrey GU2 5XH, UK

Terry M. Brooks, Shell Resarch Ltd, Sittingbourne Research Centre, Sittingbourne, Kent ME9 8AG, UK

Brian Burlinson, Genetic and Reproductive Toxicology Department, Glaxo Group Research, Ware, Hertfordshire SG12 0DJ, UK

Stephen W. Dean, Hazleton Microtest, Otley Road, Harrogate, North Yorkshire HG3 1PY, UK

Edward P. Evans, MRC Radiobiology Unit, Chilton, Didcot, Oxfordshire OX11 0RD, UK

Jack Favor, GSF-Forschungszentrum für Umwelt und Gesundheit, Institut für Säugetiergenetik, Ingolstädter Landstrasse 1, D-8042, Neuherberg, Germany

L. Michael Holmstrom, Inveresk Research International Ltd, Tranent, Edinburgh EH33 2NE, UK

Diane E. Kelly, Department of Molecular Biology and Biotechnology, The University, Sheffield, S10 2TN, UK

Steven L. Kelly, Department of Molecular Biology and Biotechnology, The University, Sheffield, S10 2TN, UK

James C. Kennelly, Zeneca plc, Central Toxicology Laboratory, Alderley Park, Macclesfield, Cheshire SK10 4TJ, UK

David J. Kirkland, Hazleton Microtest, Otley Road, Harrogate, Yorkshire HG3 1PY, UK

Philip D. Lawley, Institute of Cancer Research, The Haddow Laboratories, 15 Cotswold Road, Belmont, Sutton, Surrey SM2 5NG, UK

Paul A. Lefevre, Zeneca plc, Central Toxicology Laboratory, Alderley Park, Macclesfield, Cheshire SK10 4TJ, UK

James M. Mackay, Zeneca plc, Central Toxicology Laboratory, Alderley Park, Macclesfield, Cheshire SK10 4TJ, UK

Carl N. Martin, Hazleton Microtest, Otley Road, Harrogate, North Yorkshire HG3 1PY, UK

Ian de G. Mitchell, Smith Kline Beecham Pharmaceuticals, The Frythe, Welwyn, Hertfordshire AL6 9AR, UK

Anthony K. Palmer, Huntingdon Research Centre Ltd, PO Box 2, Huntingdon, Cambridgeshire PE18 6ES, UK

James M. Parry, Molecular Biology Research Group, School of Biological Sciences, University College of Swansea, Singleton Park, Swansea SA2 8PP, UK

David Phillips, Institute of Cancer Research, The Haddow Laboratories, 15 Cotswold Road, Belmont, Sutton, Surrey SM2 5NG, UK

Charles Tease, MRC Radiobiology Unit, Chilton, Didcot, Oxfordshire OX11 0RD, UK

Stanley Venitt, Institute of Cancer Research, The Haddow Laboratories, 15 Cotswold Road, Belmont, Sutton, Surrey SM2 5NG, UK

Philip Wilcox, Genetic and Reproductive Toxicology Department, Glaxo Group Research, Ware, Hertfordshire SG12 0DJ, UK

Ray Waters, University College of Swansea, Singleton Park, Swansea SA2 8PP, UK

LIST OF ABBREVIATIONS

2-AFF	=	N-acetyl-2-aminofluorene
4-AAF	=	N-acetyl-4-aminofluorene
ACM	=	Advisory Committee on Mutagenesis (Canada)
ANOVA	=	Analysis of variance
ASTM	=	Americam Society of Testing and Materials
ATP	=	Adenosine triphosphate
COM	=	Committee on Mutagenicity (UK)
cyt P450	=	Cytochrome P45
DHSS*	=	Department of Health and Social Security (UK)
DMSO	=	dimethyl sulphoxide
DH*	=	Department of Health (UK)
EDTA	=	ethylenediaminetetraacetic acid
EEC	=	European Economic Community
EGTA	=	ethylene glycol-bis (β-aminoethyl ether), N, N, N^1, N^1-tetraacetic acid
EPA	=	Environmental Protection Agency (USA)
GLP	=	Good Laboratory Practice
HMSO	=	Her Majesty's Stationery Office
HPLC	=	high performance liquid chromatography
IARC	=	International Agency for Research on Cancer
ip	=	intraperitoneal
JMHW	=	Japanese Ministry of Health and Welfare
JMOL	=	Japanese Ministry of Labour
MMS	=	methylmethane sulphonate
MRC	=	Medical Research Council (UK)
MTD	=	maximum tolerated dose
NDMA	=	N-nitrosodimethylamine
NQO	=	4-nitroquinoline-N-oxide

* Name changed from DHSS to DH between 1981 and 1989.

OECD = Organisation for Economic Co-operation and Development
pc = post coitum
po = per os (by mouth)
SC = synaptonemal complex
SDS = sodium dodecyl sulphate
TCA = trichloracetic acid
UDS = unscheduled DNA synthesis
UFAW = Universities Federation for Animal Welfare
UKEMS = United Kingdom Environmental Mutagen Society

1

Introduction

D. J. Kirkland

1.1 GENERAL

1.1.1 Objectives

In March 1982 the United Kingdom Environmental Mutagen Society (UKEMS) appointed a Sub-committee to report on the minimal professional criteria that should be applied to mutagenicity testing in order to meet the requirements of the UK authorities. The tests recommended in the *Guidelines for the Testing of Chemicals for Mutagenicity* which was published by the Department of Health and Social Security (DHSS, 1981) formed the basis of the first report which dealt with the most commonly used mutagenicity tests (UKEMS, 1983). Other reports followed, dealing with *Supplementary Tests* (UKEMS, 1984) and *Statistical Evaluation of Mutagenicity Test Data* (UKEMS, 1989).

One objective of the Sub-committee was to ensure that these reports reflected the current state of knowledge in the field of mutagenesis, and it was suggested that each report be examined every 5 years to consider necessary revisions. The first report on basic tests was therefore reviewed and the revised version published in 1990 (UKEMS, 1990).

Since the publication of the first report in 1983, many more guidelines, recommendations, strategies and requirements for mutagenicity testing have been proposed and written. Those with the widest impact have been from the Organisation for Economic Co-operation and Development (OECD, 1983, 1984 and 1986), The European Economic Community (EEC, 1984, 1988), the Japanese Ministry of Health and Welfare (JMHW, 1984), the Japanese Ministry of Labour (JMOL, 1979), the Health Effects Guidelines of the US Environmental Protection Agency (EPA, 1982*a*, *b*), the Canadian Advisory Committee on Mutagenesis (ACM, 1986) and the American Society of Testing and Materials (ASTM, 1987). It was important, then, that any revision of the report on the supplementary tests should take such guidelines into account.

As the expert Committee on Mutagenicity (COM) of the Department of

Health has also recently revised its 1981 recommendations (DH, 1989), it was most important that any revision of the UKEMS report on the supplementary tests should reflect these changes.

1.1.2   Terms of reference
The terms of reference of the Sub-committee since its formation in 1982 are as follows:

1. to define the minimal criteria, i.e. the minimum basic experimental design required to perform current test procedures of relevant authorities to professionally acceptable standards (with due regard to the Good Laboratory Practice Guidelines);
2. to define the criteria necessary to constitute a positive result in each of the current test procedures;
3. to define the criteria and extent of testing required to identify a material as non-mutagenic in each of the current test procedures;
4. to specify modifications to standard procedures which may be required to meet specific circumstances or to answer specific problems (e.g. procedures for testing volatile materials);
5. to prepare proposals for regular updating of the test systems and protocols as envisaged by the DH Guidelines and those of other bodies with regard to accepted technical advances supported by up-to-date and appropriate references;
6. to prepare recommendations for a framework of testing procedures subsequent to the initial battery, i.e. which supplementary test should be carried out and in what circumstances.

Terms 1. to 5. are still pertinent to the current revisions, although 6. is now superfluous in that the strategic element of the new COM recommendations addresses the framework of follow-up tests.

1.1.3   Purpose and structure of the revision
As the protocols for the basic mutagenicity tests become more demanding (UKEMS, 1990) the likelihood of discrepant results between tests increases. A mixture of positive and negative results is therefore often obtained from a selection of two or three *in vitro* tests. Supplementary testing will usually be aimed at determining whether the positive or the negative findings are the most predictive of *in vivo* hazard and are the most relevant to a safety assessment. As the science has advanced since 1984, it was therefore important to review the supplementary test recommendations at this time.

The Sub-committee consists of a Steering Group, which is representative of industrial, academic, contract research and regulatory genetic toxicologists, and a series of Working Groups. The task of assessing and reporting on each of the procedures has been undertaken by the Working Groups which each consisted of a group leader plus two to seven expert members. Only five Working Groups were established for this revision though nine were involved in the development of the first report on Supplementary Tests, published in 1984. This is because it was felt there was nothing new to add, at this time, to the recommendations made for bacterial DNA repair tests, cell transformation tests, sister chromatid exchange assays, and the three specialist areas of mutagens in food, mutagens in body fluids, and mutation assays with nitrosation products.

With the continued emphasis on *in vitro* testing in many guidelines, and the need for alternative tests when, for example, antimicrobial substances dictate the Ames test is inappropriate, it was logical to revise the recommendations for conducting yeast assays. The dominant lethal assay, which was excluded from the basic tests in the DH (1989) revisions, but is recommended for consideration when effects in germ cells are to be specially investigated, and the germ cell cytogenetics assay, have also been revised. The UDS test *in vitro* has not been revised, but the chapter presented here deals with the important *in vivo/in vitro* (or *ex vivo* as it is sometimes called) version, which has now been adequately validated and forms an important method for looking *in vivo* at tissue other than bone marrow. A new chapter on DNA binding has been added. Finally, a statistician was co-opted onto the Steering Group to review the statistical issues in light of the recent UKEMS statistics guidelines (UKEMS, 1989).

1.2   SPECIAL REQUIREMENTS
1.2.1   Safety
The safety of staff involved in the conduct of mutagenicity tests described in this and earlier reports has been a fundamental consideration of the Sub-committee. It has to be emphasised that staff should be fully trained in techniques for handling hazardous chemicals and potentially hazardous materials such as human blood.

Containment areas for chemical handling and designated areas for handling potentially infected human cells should be delineated, and operating procedures should be in place to minimise handling hazards and to deal with spills. Disposal of waste containing mutagens/carcinogens or potentially infected material also requires that pre-defined safety procedures be followed.

Details of handling precautions, disposal and spillage procedures are to be found in a number of texts for chemicals (IARC, 1979, 1980; MRC, 1981; University of Birmingham, 1980) and in certain publications for pathogens and infectious material (e.g. Advisory Committee on Dangerous Pathogens, 1984).

1.2.2   Good laboratory practice

Most industrial, all contract and some academic laboratories will be conducting mutagenicity tests to provide reports to support regulatory submissions.

Scientists in many of these laboratories will be well aware of the requirements of the Good Laboratory Practice (GLP) guidelines published by various organisations. However, not all countries operate GLP compliance programmes at this time, so before conducting mutagenicity tests to support data submissions to the UK, USA, EEC and Japan in particular, it would be wise to become familiar with the following:

- Good Laboratory Practice. The UK Compliance Programme, DOH, London, 1989.
- US Food and Drug Administration, Federal Register, 21 CFR Part 58; Good Laboratory Practice Regulations, 22 December 1978 (and its subsequent revisions).
- US Environmental Protection Agency, Federal Register, 40 CFR Part 160; Pesticide Programmes; Good Laboratory Practice Standards, 29 November 1983 (and subsequent amendment, 17 August 1989).
- OECD Principles of Good Laboratory Practice. C(81)30(final) Annex 2. 12 May 1981.
- Japanese Good Laboratory Practice Guidelines of the Pharmaceutical Affairs Bureau, Ministry of Health and Welfare; Notification of 31 March 1982 (and subsequent amendment Notification No. Yakuhatsu 870, 5 October 1988).
- Japanese Ministry of Agriculture, Forestry and Fisheries, GLP requirements on toxicological studies on pesticides; Notification 59 Nohsan No. 3850, issued by the Agricultural Production Bureau, 10 August 1984.
- EC GLP Directive 87/18/EEC. Official Journal of the EC No L15 17 January 1987.
- Japanese Ministry of International Trade and Industry, Directive 31 March 1984 (Kanpogyo No. 39 Environmental Agency, Kikyoku No. 85 MITI).

1.2.3   Technical expertise

Before embarking on any mutagenicity testing, or setting up a routine screening laboratory, it is essential that suitable experimental designs, 'baseline protocols', be selected and documented. These enable consistent methods to be developed for every phase of each study, which are critical factors in successful testing. For this to occur, staff should be thoroughly trained in both the theoretical and practical aspects of the methods they will use, if necessary by seeking (and taking) advice from investigators with proven experience in the field. Staff involved in testing should be able to demonstrate their proficiency, for example, by correctly classifying the mutagenicity of a range of reference compounds.

1.3 TEST MATERIALS

1.3.1 Description

Testing substances 'blind' is to be strongly discouraged for routine testing, and is especially inappropriate when supplementary testing.

Details of the test material should be obtained from the supplier. It is important that the testing facility obtains as much information as possible including, where appropriate:

- source
- batch number
- purity
- known impurities
- physical form and appearance
- chemical structure
- solubility
- reactivity in aqueous and non-aqueous solvents or vehicles
- stability to temperature, pH and light
- storage conditions
- stability of solutions to temperature, pH and light
- adverse effects on man

If the full chemical name or CAS number can be obtained, and other relevant information such as colour index number for dyes, etc, this information should be reported. If the test material is a volatile liquid or gas, its boiling point and vapour pressure should be given. The investigator should check the appearance of characteristics of the test material on receipt against the supplier's description, and make an independent record of the physical appearance and conditions of storage.

1.3.2 Handling

Unless reliable data are available to the contrary, test substances should be handled as if they were toxic to man, unstable, and sensitive to light and heat. When testing substances which are destined for topical use, and/or where there is reason to suspect that the substances (e.g. sun-screens) may be photo-activated, either by design or incidentally, special controls need to be included or supplementary experiments should be performed to determine the effects of light of the appropriate wavelengths.

1.3.3   Preparation of solutions/suspensions

Whenever possible, solutions or suspensions of test substances should be freshly prepared immediately before each experiment, and unused portions should not be re-used unless there are appropriate stability data. When testing up to the limit of solubility in the test system, it may be necessary to examine a selection of solvents or suspending agents, and dilutions thereof, before deciding the best scheme. Maximum solubility is defined as the highest concentration at which there is no visible precipitation. In all cases, however, the investigator must ensure that concentrations of organic solvents remain within levels tolerated by the test organism, and have regard for the fact that use of an unusual solvent may necessitate inclusion of untreated controls, or preliminary investigations to ensure the solvent does not adversely affect spontaneous mutation/aberration frequencies or viability.

It may be wise to check the effect an unusual solvent may have on pH and osmolality in the light of the artefactual positive results that may be a consequence of such changes (Brusick, 1987).

If positive results are obtained and a known impurity that gives rise to some concern (e.g. because of its structure) is present in the test substance, it is recommended that, whenever possible, the impurity be assayed for mutagenicity at concentrations equivalent to those which would have been present in the positive concentration range of the parent test material used in the initial assay. If a mixture is to be tested, this should be stated. Since many mixtures are difficult to define chemically, details of their preparation should be provided. If it is known that one or more of the starting materials is a major constituent, it may be advisable to assay this in parallel with the mixture.

1.3.4   Special approaches

The comments above all apply to chemical test materials. If the test agent is physical in nature (e.g. radiation of various types) a full description of the source, distance from source, dose rate, time of exposure, means of exposure (i.e. with or without lid, or medium; static or roller bottles, etc) and, preferably, a measure of the delivered 'dose' should be given.

1.4   POSITIVE CONTROLS
1.4.1   Choice of chemical(s)

The chemicals most widely used as positive controls are well documented in the literature, and often recommended in guidelines such as those of OECD (1983, 1984, 1986). The chemicals chosen should be those which the investigator has shown to act reproducibly in the system under test, and which identify satisfactory metabolic activation conditions, or discriminate between different strains or sexes or response times. Different controls should, for example, be used in non-activation and activation parts of an *in vitro* test.

It is often recommended that additional class-related positive controls should be used, for example hydrazines when hydrazine-containing drugs are under test, as recommended by Ashby and Purchase (1979). Such procedures are to be encouraged where appropriate, but it is recognised that, with many compounds, it may not be possible to identify a class-related mutagen.

1.4.2   Choice of concentrations

It is recommended that, prior to a testing programme, each laboratory should construct dose–response curves for each positive control mutagen in each test system, and accumulate a database of historical positive (and negative) control responses. This will determine the sensitivity of each assay in their hands. The test concentration chosen for each reference mutagen should then be set at a level which is close to the limits of detection and which would be expected to test the performance and resolution of the assay, rather than at a level which will always give highly positive responses irrespective of the sensitivity of the assay on any given occasion. An alternative, and equally acceptable, approach to utilising a low dose of potent mutagen, is to utilise a moderate dose of a weak mutagen. Either way, the investigator must be able to demonstrate that the test system is consistently able to detect small increases in mutant/aberration frequency.

1.5   PRESENTATION OF RESULTS
1.5.1   Minimum data to be presented

The description of the experimental design should be detailed enough to allow independent replication of the assay. Precise details of the protocol should be provided; if a published protocol was used this should be referred to, and any deviations from it should be clearly documented. The source and the method of preparation of any exogenous metabolic activation system should be given, together with details of any inducers which were used.

For *in vivo* studies the supplier of animals should be identified, together with information on strain and sex used in the test, and the quality of drinking water, diet and bedding.

For regulatory purposes, 'raw' data should be provided, including results obtained for negative and positive controls. Such data should always be given in addition to mutation frequencies or other transformations. Presentation of raw data allows independent statistical evaluation. Historical control data should also be presented to permit the results to be viewed in the light of the longer-term experiences of the testing laboratory.

1.5.2   Data processing

Data analysis methods should be carefully documented or referenced. UKEMS working groups have published their own recommendations for analysis of data obtained from some of the assays discussed herein (UKEMS, 1989).

1.5.3   Publication of data

Publication of data in scientific journals is strongly encouraged wherever possible. Not only does this ensure that robust protocols are used to generate high quality, reliable data, but it enables others to evaluate the performance of various protocols (which is critical in the development of testing strategies), and to repeat the work independently. The peer review process is an important control element in ensuring the quality of data.

1.6   REFERENCES

ACM (1986). *Guidelines on the Use of Mutagenicity Tests in the Toxicological Evaluation of Chemicals.* A Report of the DNH & W/DOE Environmental Contaminants Advisory Committee on Mutagenesis. National Health and Welfare and Environment, Canada.

Advisory Committee on Dangerous Pathogens (1984). *Categorisation of Pathogens according to Hazard and Categories of Containment.*

Ashby, J. & Purchase, I. F. H. (1979). The selection of appropriate chemical class controls for use with short-term tests for potential carcinogenicity. *Annals of Occupational Hygiene*, **20**, 297–301.

ASTM (1987). R. W. Naismith, ed. Guidelines for minimal criteria of acceptability for selected short-term assays for genotoxicity. *Mutation Research*, **189**, 81–183.

Brusick, D. (1987). Implications of treatment condition-induced genotoxicity for chemical screening and data interpretation. *Mutation Research*, **189**, 1–6.

DHSS (1981). Guidelines for Testing of Chemicals for Mutagenicity. Prepared by the Committee on Mutagenicity of Chemicals in Food, Consumer Products and the Environment. Department of Health and Social Security. *Report on Health and Social Subjects No. 24.* Her Majesty's Stationery Office, London.

DH (1989). Guidelines for Testing of Chemicals for Mutagenicity. Prepared by the Committee on Mutagenicity of Chemicals in Food, Consumer Products and the Environment. Department of Health. *Report on Health and Social Subjects No. 35.*

EEC (1984). Methods for the determination of physico-chemical properties, toxicity and ecotoxicity: Annex V to Directive 67/548/EEC. *Official Journal of the European Communities No. L251*, 131–45.

EEC (1988). Methods for the determination of toxicity and ecotoxicity. *Official Journal of the European Communities No. L133*, 55–87.

EPA (1982a). *Health Effects Test Guidelines.* Office of Toxic Substances. Environmental Protection Agency, Washington, USA, August 1982.

EPA (1982b). *Pesticide Assessment Guidelines, Subdivision F Hazard Evaluation: Human and Domestic Animals.* Office of Pesticides and Toxic

Substances. Environmental Protection Agency, Washington, USA. October 1982.

IARC (1979). Some halogenated hydrocarbons. *IARC Monographs on the Evaluation of the Carcinogenic Risk of Chemicals to Humans, 20.* International Agency for Research on Cancer, Lyon, pp. 85–106.

IARC (1980). *Laboratory Decontamination and Destruction of Aflatoxins B¹, B₂, G₁, G²* in *Laboratory Wastes.* Ed. M. Castegnaro, D. C. Hunt, E. B. Sansone, P. L. Schuller, M. G. Siriwardana, G. M. Telling, H. P. von Egmond and E. A. Walker. IARC Scientific Publications. International Agency for Research on Cancer, Lyon.

JMHW (1984). *Information on the Guidelines of Toxicity Studies Required for applications for approval to Manufacture (Import) Drugs (Part 1).* Notification No. 118 of the Pharmaceutical Affairs Bureau, Ministry of Health and Welfare, Japan.

JMOL (1979). *On the Standards of the Mutagenicity Test Using Micro-Organisms. The Labour Safety and Hygiene Law.* The Labour Standard Bureau, Ministry of Labour, Japan.

MRC (1981). *Guidelines for Work with Chemical Carcinogens in Medical Research Council Establishments.* Medical Research Council, London.

OECD (1983). *OECD Guideline for Testing of Chemicals, Genetic Toxicology, No. 471–474.* Organisation for Economic Co-operation and Development, Paris, 26 May 1983.

OECD (1984). *OECD Guideline for Testing of Chemicals, Genetic Toxicology, No. 475–478.* 4 April 1984.

OECD (1986). *OECD Guideline for Testing of Chemicals, Genetic Toxicology, No. 479–485.* 23 October 1986.

UKEMS (1983). *UKEMS Sub-committee on Guidelines for Mutagenicity Testing. Report. Part I. Basic Test Battery.* Ed. B. J. Dean. United Kingdom Environmental Mutagen Society, Swansea.

UKEMS (1984). *UKEMS Sub-committee on Guidelines for Mutagenicity Testing. Report. Part II. Supplementary Tests.* Ed. B. J. Dean. United Kingdom Environmental Mutagen Society, Swansea.

UKEMS (1989). *UKEMS Sub-committee on Guidelines for Mutagenicity Testing. Report. Part III. Statistical Evaluation of Mutagenicity Test Data.* Ed. D. J. Kirkland. Cambridge University Press.

UKEMS (1990). *Basic Mutagenicity Tests: UKEMS Recommended Procedures.* Ed. D. J. Kirkland. Cambridge University Press. Cambridge.

University of Birmingham (1980). *Rules and Notes of Guidance for the Use of Chemical Carcinogens in the University.* The University of Birmingham, Birmingham, UK.

2

Genotoxicity studies using yeast cultures

T. M. Brooks   D. E. Kelly   S. L. Kelly
I. de G. Mitchell   J. M. Parry   P. Wilcox

2.1   INTRODUCTION

In contrast to the expansion in the use of yeast in molecular biology, there has been little change in most areas of yeast mutagenicity testing over the last few years. This is due, in part, to the advances made in mammalian cell assays, which have restricted the role/advantages of using yeast in testing chemicals for mutagenic activity.

Factors favouring the use of yeast cultures in genotoxicity studies are the number of modifications that are to be found in the published data relating to genetic endpoints, treatment protocols and activation systems (Zimmermann, Mayer & Scheel, 1984a; Parry & Parry, 1984). They may also be used as an alternative to bacterial assays for testing anti-bacterial agents to avoid bacterial-specific effects (Mitchell et al., 1980) and to enable adequate concentrations to be tested.

The most commonly used yeast in genotoxicity studies is the budding yeast *Saccharomyces cerevisiae*. This physiologically robust organism tolerates pH values between 3 and 9 and survives at temperatures from freezing to above 40 °C. Growth can occur over a temperature range of 18 °C to 40 °C, but is optimal at 28 °C using a carbon source such as glucose.

Haploid yeast strains of the *a* and the ∝ mating type and diploids heterozygous and homozygous for mating type may be cultivated continuously in the vegetative stage in/on both liquid and solid medium with the appropriate medium changes. In mixed cultures of *a* and ∝ haploid cells mating takes place to produce heterozygous *a*/∝ diploids and such diploids may be induced to undergo meiosis in exhausted medium or on potassium acetate sporulation medium. Meiosis results in a reduction division leading to the production of highly resistant 4 spored asci, made up of 2*a* and 2∝ spores. On inoculation into fresh nutrient medium, such spores give rise to vegetative cultures of both haploid mating types.

2.2   GENETIC ENDPOINTS

The major advantage of yeast for genotoxicity studies is the comprehensive range of genetic endpoints that may be assayed. These include:

1. gene mutation in chromosomal and mitochondrial genes;
2. recombination between and within genes and within chromosomes;
3. chromosomal aneuploidy during both mitosis and meiosis.

2.2.1   Gene mutation

A variety of forward and reverse mutation systems have been used with haploid, and occasionally with diploid, yeast strains.

2.2.1.1   *Forward mutation*

The system of longest standing is the mutation of 'red colony' phenotype adenine (*ade*1 and *ade*2) auxotrophs to 'white colony' mutants (Roman, 1956). Here mutations in any (of five) loci in the adenine synthetic pathway that precede the production of the red pigment may result in the generation of white colonies. The problem with this system is that it is non-selective so that about 20 000 colonies need to be scored to justify a negative conclusion (Brusick, 1980).

Other systems involve mutation from sensitivity to resistance to substances toxic to yeasts. The most popular of these is mutation to canavanine resistance (*can*^{r}) which is thought to result from arginine permease deficiency (Grenson *et al.*, 1966; Thacker, 1974). Another well-validated system is mutation to cycloheximide resistance (*cyh*^{r}) (Brusick, 1972) which involves an alteration of ribosome structure. Initially, it was thought that this system would only detect base substitutions; however, recent work has demonstrated that frameshift agents are detected as well (Rees *et al.*, 1989; Mitchell & Gilbert, 1991). Finally, a promising system is mutation to D,L-α-amino-adipic acid resistance (*ada*^{r}) (Mitchell & Gilbert, 1991) based on the method used for selection of *lys*2 and *lys*5 auxotrophy (Chattoo *et al.*, 1979). It should be noted that, in most forward mutation systems, a period of growth under non-selective conditions is required before exposure to the toxic agent (Lawrence, 1982); in the case of canavanine resistance a growth period of at least 11 hours is required (Lemontt, 1977).

2.2.1.2   *Reverse (point) mutation*

The best validated reverse mutation system is with the multiply marked, auxotrophic, haploid strain XV185-14C (Mehta & von Borstel, 1981). Base substitution can be detected by site-specific reversion or suppression of the ochre nonsense mutations *ade*2-1, *arg*4-17, *trp*5-48 *and lys*1-1. The *his*1-7 locus is a mis-sense mutation reverted mainly by second site mutations, whilst the *hom3*-10 mutation is thought to be a frameshift (von Borstel & Quah, 1973).

In the diploid strain, D7, reversion of the homozygous *ilv*1-92 locus can be assayed (Zimmermann, Kern & Rasenberger, 1975). However, this assay only detects a limited range of chemical mutagens, i.e. those that induce base pair substitution and is therefore unsuitable for routine screening.

2.2.1.3   *General aspects of gene mutation assays*

Yeast gene mutation assays have generally performed well in collaborative trials, which have evaluated mutagenicity/carcinogenicity correlations (Mehta & von Borstel, 1981). However, they tend to be insensitive to water-insoluble polycyclic or heterocyclic aromatic compounds which are carcinogenic in animals, induce frameshift mutations in the Ames test and usually need microsomal activation. Attempts to improve sensitivity with permeabilizing treatments (Boguslawski, 1985; Mitchell & Gilbert, 1985) or with permeable mutants (Morita *et al.*, 1989) have met with only limited success. It would seem that forward mutation assays are more sensitive to such agents than reverse mutation systems (Mitchell & Gilbert, 1985, 1991) and some strains are more sensitive than others. Overall, results suggest that the cycloheximide resistance system is the most sensitive assay, particularly using minimal agar and low levels (0.5 μg per ml) of cycloheximide (Mitchell & Gilbert, 1991).

2.2.1.4   *Mutation of extra-chromosomal genes*

The induction of 'petite' mutation in the autonomously replicating mitochondria of yeast by chemicals has been studied for many years (Ephrussi, 1950). The DNA organisation in mitochondria is prokaryotic rather than eukaryotic and these organelles are non-essential in *S. cerevisiae*. The main reason why this system has not achieved wide acceptance as a genotoxicity assay is that the significance of a positive finding is not clear. A further problem is that early results with this system were not reproducible (Gilberg & Aman, 1971; Kilbey & Zetterberg, 1973). Nevertheless, some workers have claimed that the system has a special relevance to carcinogenicity, see Section 2.3.3.6 (Patel & Wilkie, 1982).

2.2.2   **Recombination**

In eukaryotic cells, genetic exchanges between homologous chromo-somes are generally confined to a specialised stage of meiotic cell division which in yeast occurs during the process of sporulation. However, in yeast, recombinational events may also be detected during mitotic division, although the spontaneous frequency is generally at least 1000 times less than that observed during meiosis. Sporulating yeast cultures may be used to study the rate of both spontaneous and induced meiotic recombination, but it is generally the mitotic events that are of practical value in genotoxicity studies. Mitotic recombination can be detected in yeast both between genes (or more generally between a gene and the centromere) and within genes. The former event is called mitotic crossing-over and generates reciprocal products, whereas the latter event is most frequently non-reciprocal and is called gene conversion. Crossing-over is generally assayed by the production of recessive homozygous colonies or sectors produced in a heterozygous strain, whereas gene conversion is assayed by the production of prototrophic revertants produced in a hetero-allelic strain carrying two different defective alleles of the same gene. Mitotic gene conversion can functionally be distinguished from point mutation due to the elevated levels of prototrophy produced in heteroallelic strains compared to homoallelic strains (carrying two copies of the same mutation).

The value of assays for mitotic recombination in yeast in genotoxicity studies stems from the observations that both events are elevated by exposure to genetically active chemicals. These increases are produced in a non-specific manner, i.e. levels are increased by all types of mutagens irrespective of their mode of action. Thus the primary advantage of assaying for the induction of mitotic recombination is that the events involved are reflective of the cell's response to a wide spectrum of genetic damage. A variety of suitable strains of *Saccharomyces cerevisiae* have been constructed for use in genotoxicity testing. However, for the purpose of this report we will confine ourselves to those most frequently utilised and convenient for use.

Mitotic gene conversion may be assayed using selective medium in the diploid *Saccharomyces cerevisiae* strain D4 (Zimmermann, 1975). The genotype of D4 is shown in Fig. 2.1.

ade2-2, ade2-1, trp5-12 and *trp5-27* are heteroalleles, i.e. defective at different sites of the *ADE2* and *TRP5* loci respectively. Mitotic gene conversion can result in the production of prototrophic colonies carrying one wild

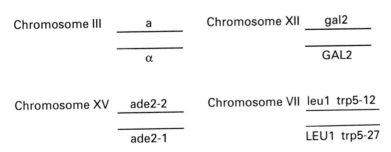

Fig. 2.1.

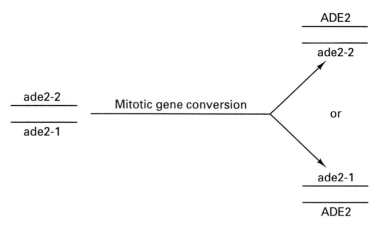

Fig. 2.2.

type allele, which is sufficient to allow growth on selective medium lacking either tryptophan or adenine (Fig. 2.2).

The D4 strain has been extensively used in the study of genotoxic chemicals (Zimmermann *et al.*, 1984*b*) and has proved to be a valuable tool. However, the use of this strain is limited by the relatively high spontaneous reversion frequencies of the *ADE2* marker, which means that if this locus is to be used, cultures with a low spontaneous frequency of prototrophy must be selected prior to chemical treatment. Mitotic gene conversion may also be assayed in the strain JD1 (Sharp & Parry, 1981) which is additionally capable of simultaneously detecting mitotic crossing-over on chromosome XV. The genotype of JD1 is shown in Fig. 2.3.

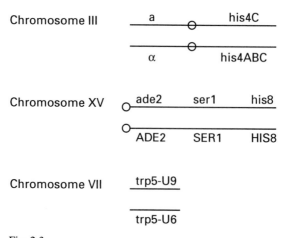

Fig. 2.3

his4C, his4ABC, trp5-U9 and trp5-U6 are heteroalleles at the *HIS4* and *TRP5* loci respectively. They undergo mitotic gene conversion to produce prototrophic colonies carrying one wild-type allele, which allows growth on selective medium lacking either tryptophan or histidine. Mitotic crossing-over may be assayed by the production of red colonies or sectors homozygous for *ade-2* and the markers distal on chromosome XV (Fig. 2.4).

JD1 thus allows the assay of mitotic gene conversion at two separate loci and also detects one of the possible homozygous chromosome combinations produced by mitotic crossing-over (but not both reciprocal products). The strain has been selected for its inability to undergo sporulation and is thus suitable for long treatment times. Protocols are also available for the use of this strain under conditions which produce optimal expression of the yeast cytochrome P450 (Kelly & Parry, 1983).

A particularly convenient multipurpose strain of *Saccharomyces cerevisiae* is D7 (Zimmermann, 1975) which carries a set of genetic markers which allow the simultaneous assay of mitotic crossing-over, gene conversion and point mutation (Fig. 2.5).

trp5-12 and trp5-27 are heteroalleles of the *TRP5* locus and undergo mitotic gene conversion to produce prototrophic colonies carrying one wild-type allele which allows for growth on selective medium lacking tryptophan. ade2-40 is a completely inactive allele of *ADE2* which produces deep red colonies whereas ade2-119 is a leaky allele causing accumulation of only a small amount of pigment and thus producing pink colonies. In heteroallelic diploids, the ade2-40 and ade2-119 alleles complement to give rise to white adenine independent colonies. Mitotic crossing-over in D7 may give rise to the

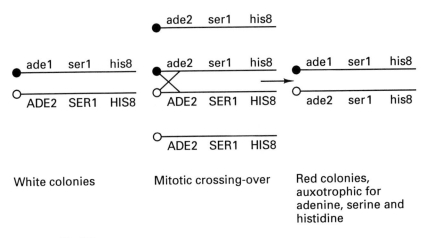

White colonies   Mitotic crossing-over   Red colonies, auxotrophic for adenine, serine and histidine

Fig. 2.4.

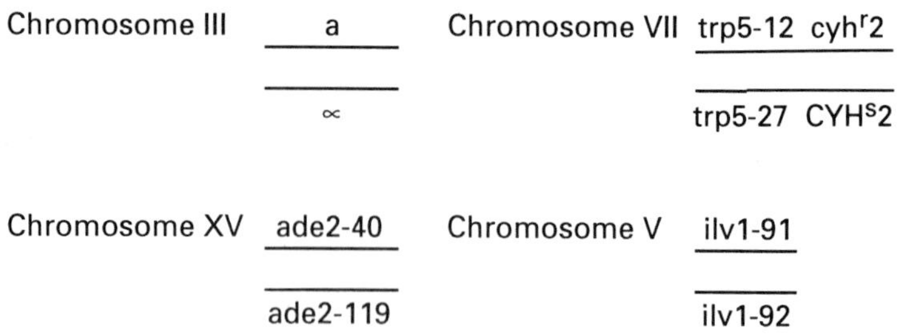

Chromosome III
a
∝
Chromosome VII
trp5-12 cyhr2
trp5-27 CYHS2
Chromosome XV
ade2-40
ade2-119
Chromosome V
ilv1-91
ilv1-92

Fig. 2.5

production of cells homoallelic for the *ade*2 mutations and thus lead to the observation of both red and pink reciprocal products (Fig. 2.6).

Thus the frequency of induced reciprocal mitotic crossing-over can be unambiguously confirmed in D7 by the visual observation of twin-sectored colonies. Mitotic crossing-over may also be assayed in D7 by the use of the recessive cycloheximide resistant cyh^{r}_{2} allele on chromosome VII. Crossing-over between *CYH*2 and the centromere of chromosome VII results in the production of colonies which are capable of growth on medium containing cycloheximide (Kunz, Barclay & Haynes, 1980) (Fig. 2.7).

A non-sporulating derivative of D7, i.e. D7-144 has been isolated, which is suitable for use over long treatment times (Mehta & von Borstel, 1985). The diploid strain BZ_{34} (Fogel & Mortimer, 1969) has also been used to assay for gene conversion (Sankaranarayanan & Murthy, 1979). It has non-complementing mutant alleles at the arginosuccinase locus (*arg*4) which results in a growth requirement for arginine.

An interesting new strain which has recently become available is RS112 developed by Schiestl and his colleagues (Schiestl, Igarashi & Hastings, 1988). This strain has been constructed to allow the measurement of the induction of intrachromosomal recombination, an event which may occur within chromosomes and may lead to deletion of genetic material. In the

ade2-40
ade2-119
ade2-40
ade2-40
ade2-119
ade2-119
ade2-40
ade2-40
ade2-119
ade2-119
Red colonies
Pink colonies

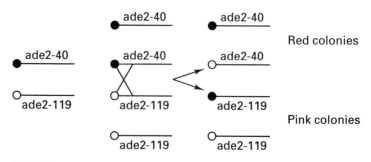

Fig. 2.6.

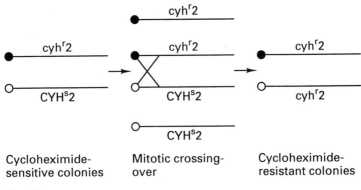

Cycloheximide-sensitive colonies   Mitotic crossing-over   Cycloheximide-resistant colonies

Fig. 2.7

diploid RS112, intrachromosomal recombination may be monitored in chromosome XV, a copy of which contains a deletion of the *HIS*-3 gene (his 3 – Δ 200), whereas the other homologue carries a *HIS*-3 gene which has been disrupted by the incorporation of the plasmid pRS6. Plasmid pRS6 contains the DNA sequences for the plasmid pBR322, the yeast leu-2 gene and a fragment of the *HIS*-3 gene which allows integration into the *HIS*-3 gene of a recipient yeast strain. The essential features of chromosome XV of RS112 are shown in Fig. 2.8.

The induction of intrachromosomal recombination within chromosome XV results in the deletion of the plasmid, which may lead to the reconstitution of a functional *HIS*-3 gene as shown in Fig. 2.9. This event has been classified as a deletion (DEL) event by Schiestl and co-workers (Schiestl, 1989).

The complete genotype of RS112 is: Mat a/∝, *ura3*-52/*ura3*-52, *leu2*-3,112/*leu2*-Δ98, *trp5*-27/*TRP*-5, *arg4*-3/*ARG4*, *ade2*-40/*ade2*-101, *ilv* 1-92/*ILV1*, *HIS*-3::pRS6/*his3*-Δ200, *LYS2*/*lys*-801. The presence of two heteroalleles *ade2*-40/*ade2*-101 on chromosome XV also allows the simultaneous measurement of mitotic gene conversion.

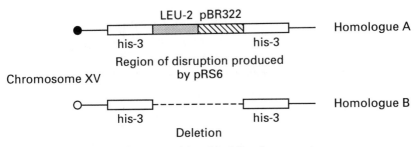

Strain RS112 requiring histidine for growth

Fig. 2.8.

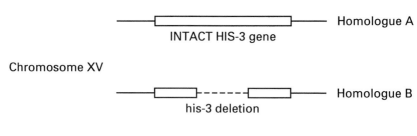

Fig. 2.9.

The main reason for the current interest in the use of strain RS112 is the report (Schiestl, 1989) that DEL events are induced by chemical carcinogens that are not routinely detectable in the standard bacterial mutagenicity assays or in yeast assays measuring mitotic gene conversion. If these data can be reproduced, the measurement of DEL events may lead to a major increase in the potential use of yeast cultures in the detection of chemical carcinogens. However, we must express our reservations over the very high concentration ranges in which some of these responses were produced. The relevance of the DEL responses observed at such treatment concentrations must be question-able, as in most cases we would not recommend the testing of chemicals in yeast at concentrations above 5 mg per ml (see Section 2.3.7). At this stage, we are unable to recommend routine studies with this strain until further validation work has been performed.

2.2.3   Aneuploidy

Abnormal chromosome segregation leading to the production of numerical chromosome aberrations may be detected in yeast by genetic means using appropriate yeast strains (for review, see Resnick, Mayer & Zimmermann, 1986). Reasonably well-validated assays are available for detecting and quantifying the induction of monosomy (chromosome loss) during mitotic cell division from the $2n$ to the $2n-1$ condition, and the production of disomy (chromosome gain) and diploidisation in spores produced during meiotic cell division (sporulation).

Prior to 1984, most published work on chemically-induced mitotic aneuploidy in yeast used the strain D6, described by Parry and Zimmermann (1976). The genotype of *Saccharomyces cerevisiae* D6 is shown in Fig. 2.10.

This strain forms red colonies because of the presence of *ade*2-40 in a homozygous condition and is sensitive to the presence of cycloheximide in

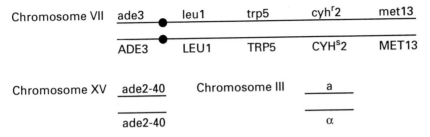

Fig. 2.10.

the medium because the *cyh*ʳ2 resistance allele is recessive. The loss of the chromosome homologue carrying the dominant wild-type allele of this group of linked markers results in cells that form white (due to the expression of *ade*3), cycloheximide resistant colonies (due to the expression of the selective cyhʳ₂ marker) that also express the markers *leu*1, *trp*5 and *met*13.

Zimmermann and Scheel (1984) developed a similar strain, D61.M, and this has now largely superseded D6 for the study of mitotic aneuploidy in yeast (Albertini, Friederich & Würgler, 1988; Whittaker *et al.*, 1989, 1990*a*). The relevant markers in D61.M are as in Fig. 2.11.

Like D6, D61.M forms red colonies (due to the *ade*2-40 marker) and is sensitive to cycloheximide. Loss of the copy of chromosome VII carrying the wild-type alleles results in simultaneous expression of the *ade*6, *leu*1 and *cyr*ʳ₂ alleles. Such cells will give rise to white colonies (since *ade*6 blocks the adenine synthetic pathway prior to *ade*2 block) which will grow on cycloheximide-containing medium and have a growth requirement for leucine. The main theoretical advantage of D61.M over D6 is that the *ade*6 marker

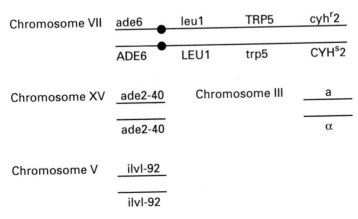

Fig. 2.11.

is much closer to the centromere than *ade*3, and thus generation of the homozygous condition by mitotic crossing over is less likely. Nevertheless, it is still important to check that suspected aneuploid colonies have simultaneously acquired a growth requirement for leucine, since it is possible to generate white, cycloheximide-resistant colonies by double crossover events, or a combination of mitotic recombination, point mutation and chromosome deletion.

When scoring the cycloheximide plates for aneuploid clones, it may be noted that some compounds increase the number of red cycloheximide-resistant colonies. Such colonies can arise by mitotic crossing-over, mitotic gene conversion, point mutation or chromosome deletion affecting the cyh_2 locus, and an increase in their frequency provides an indication that the compound possesses genotoxic activity. In the event of a large increase in red cyclo-heximide colonies, the possibility that even confirmed aneuploid clones (i.e. white, $cyh_2{}^r$, *leu*⁻) could be due to multiple recombinogenic or mutational events should be considered (Mayer & Goin, 1989). An indication of a compound's genotoxic potential can also be obtained by scoring for reverse mutation at the homozygous *ilv*1-92 marker, which responds to base pair substitution mutagens, although it would be more usual to monitor such events in a different strain, e.g. D7. The induction of petite mutations in pre-existing cyh^r cells can also cause confusion when scoring for aneuploid clones (Mayer, Goin & Zimmerman, 1986). This is because, unlike 'grande' cells, petite mutants do not appear to accumulate the red pigment which is normally produced as a consequence of the *ade*2 block.

Although strains D6 and D61.M were designed to detect mitotic aneuploidy involving chromosome VII, tetrad analysis has revealed that less than 10% of presumed aneuploid clones are in fact monosomic for this chromosome (Zimmermann *et al.*, 1985*a*). The majority of presumed monosomes have been shown to carry *two* copies of the marked chromosome VII (i.e. they are homozygous for all the nutritional markers). The most likely explanation for this is that an initial aneuploid event occurs, involving loss of the wild-type homologue, but during subsequent growth of this cell/clone there is selective advantage for cells in which the diploid state has been restored, presumably by a second aneuploid event (Whittaker *et al.*, 1989). Some support for this mechanism has been provided by Resnick, Skaanild & Nilsson-Tillgren (1989) using a strain with a divergent pair of chromosomes III.

A number of other yeast strains have been described in the literature which allow the detection of mitotic aneuploidy; these include BR1669 (Rockmill & Fogel, 1988; Whittaker *et al.*, 1988; 1990*b*), LBL1 (Esposito *et al.*, 1982), g 632 and g 551 (Kunz & Haynes, 1982) and XD72 and XD79 (Dixon, 1983). Of these, BR1669 is probably the most interesting since, unlike all the other strains discussed, it allows the detection of chromosome gain (2n + 1) and can be used to study both mitotic and meiotic events. However, only a limited number of compounds have been tested in this strain and at present it is not considered to be sufficiently validated for recommendation in this document.

In order to study chromosome malsegregation during meiosis, Sora, Lucchini & Magni (1982), Sora, Crippa & Lucchini (1983), Sora (1985), Sora & Magni (1988) have developed a strain DIS13 that carries multiple recessive, auxotrophic markers on chromosome V; the full genotype is shown in Fig. 2.12.

During meiosis of strain DIS13, spores are produced which carry multiple auxotrophic requirements (i.e. of the defective alleles on the homologues of chromosome V) and are unable to grow on minimal medium. However, spores disomic for chromosome V (*n* + 1) and diploid spores (*2n*) are capable of growth on minimal medium and their frequency may be determined by the use of the appropriate selective medium. Unsporulated diploid vegetative cells may be eliminated by the use of appropriate enzyme and detergent treatment (Garde, 1986) and disomic and diploid spores distinguished by the behaviour of the markers on chromosome VII, XV and III.

In view of the failure of yeast systems to detect some potent mammalian aneugens, e.g. colchicine and vinblastine (Parry *et al.*, 1990), it is not recommended that these systems be used as primary screens for the detection of aneugens. Rather, such systems offer a means of investigating mechanisms of chemical action and studying the relationship between aneuploidy and induced recombination in a simple eukaryote, where the genetic consequences of such events can be comprehensively analysed.

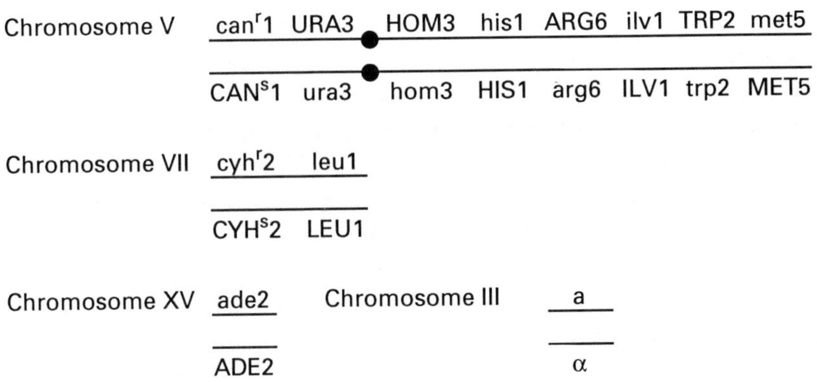

Chromosome V	can^r1 URA3	HOM3	his1	ARG6	ilv1	TRP2	met5
	CAN^s1 ura3	hom3	HIS1	arg6	ILV1	trp2	MET5

Chromosome VII	cyh^r2	leu1
	CYH^s2	LEU1

Chromosome XV	ade2		Chromosome III	a
	ADE2			α

Fig. 2.12.

2.3   THE PROCEDURE

2.3.1   General

Protocols for yeast mutagenicity assays tend to be more varied than for many other genotoxicity assays. This should not necessarily be regarded as a disadvantage, since it allows the experimenter to select treatment conditions which are most suitable for the chemical being examined. For this strategy to be successful, detailed knowledge of the physical properties of the test compound and its stability under different conditions is required. Wherever possible, this information should be obtained and taken into account in designing the experiments. The medium and reagents used in yeast systems and the general procedures for mutagenicity assays with yeast have been reviewed by Zimmermann (1973*a*, 1975) and Parry and Parry (1984). The most popular protocols for yeast mutagenicity assays are so called 'treat and plate' methods. Cells are exposed to the test chemical in liquid medium and after a prescribed treatment time, washed free of chemical and plated onto appropriate medium to assess induced genetic events and cell survival. The data are then usually expressed as mutants or convertants per surviving cell (normally per 10^6 cells).

Plate incorporation methods similar to the Salmonella/microsome assay (Ames, McCann & Yamasaki, 1975) have been used with yeast cells (Brusick, 1980) but they appear to be less sensitive than liquid treatment methods (Shahin & von Borstel, 1978; Jagannath, Vultaggio & Brusick, 1981). Also, as these methods do not allow assessment of cell viability, they can provide only semi-quantitative results. Spot tests have been used with yeast assays (see, for example, Brusick & Zeiger, 1972) but these are generally insensitive and are not recommended. Yeasts have also been used in fluctuation assays (Parry, 1977) but the method has received only limited use.

2.3.2   Stationary phase versus growing cells

There has been some debate as to the relative merits of treating exponentially growing or stationary phase cells. Growing cells have been found to be generally more sensitive to chemical mutagens. In the 'paired compound trial' (de Serres & Ashby, 1981), the use of growing cells allowed the detection of certain mutagens which were classified as negative using stationary phase cells. Other observations that growing cells are more sensitive than stationary cells to specific mutagenic agents have been made by Shahin (1975), Davies & Parry (1976), Parry, Davies & Evans (1976), Moore (1978) and Callen (1981). However, we cannot recommend the use of growing cells only, because with certain compounds stationary phase cells are more sensitive (for example, see Shahin, 1975; Zetterberg & Bostrom, 1981).

The use of growing cells for mutagenicity assays presents certain problems not encountered with stationary phase cells. Logarithmically growing yeast cells in liquid medium usually form clusters or chains which, when plated onto complete agar medium, may give rise to only one discernible colony. On selective medium, however, each cell in the cluster is capable of growing into a revertant colony and, as mutations are rare events, it is unlikely that two cells in the same cluster will be mutated. These clustering effects can therefore give rise to problems in estimating the mutation/conversion frequency. However, when yeast cells enter the stationary phase of growth, the clusters generally fall apart into single cells thus eliminating the problem. Treatment of growing cells can also give problems with pH control. Growing cells excrete acid into the medium and rapidly lower the pH; this may affect the mutagenic activity of certain chemicals.

Another problem is that components of yeast complete growth medium, such as yeast extract and peptones, can act as scavengers for reactive species and reduce their effective concentration in the treatment mix. This can be particularly important with chemicals whose activity is dependent on the generation of short-lived metabolites by an exogenous activation system. With stationary phase cells, treatment is usually carried out in simple chemical buffers so that scavenging and pH effects are not a problem. Finally, the use of growing cells with systems based on reversion to prototrophy increases the possibility of selective effects which can give rise to false positive results (see Section 2.3.6).

Despite these disadvantages, because of their increased sensitivity, the use of growing cells is still recommended for testing compounds of unknown activity. Fortunately, methods have been developed which minimise some of the problems. These will be discussed in the following section.

2.3.3 Treatment protocols with yeast mutagenicity assays

The most widely used assay system for screening chemicals for genetic activity in yeast is the induction of mitotic gene conversion. A large number of compounds have been examined in gene conversion systems and the endpoint seems to provide a sensitive, non-specific measurement of induced genetic damage (Zimmermann, 1971; Murthy, 1979; de Serres & Ashby, 1981). Protocols for this assay will therefore be considered in detail. Methods of treatment with test systems which measure other genetic endpoints are essentially the same but the method of scoring may differ. It is recommended that all studies are performed both in the presence and in the absence of an exogenous metabolic activation system.

2.3.3.1 *Mitotic gene conversion*

The following recommendations apply to systems which measure induced mitotic gene conversion by the production of prototrophic colonies in heteroallelic, auxotrophic strains. The experimental phase usually extends over 2 days. Treatment bottles are prepared on day 1, incubation with the test compound is carried out overnight, and the cells are washed and plated on day 2. The plates are then scored after an appropriate growth period.

(a)   *Treatment of growing cells*

The selected strain should be grown up in complete broth or on complete agar plates and then the cells (preferably from a single colony if this gives sufficient cells) resuspended in isotonic saline or a suitable buffer. This suspension should be used to inoculate yeast minimal broth supplemented with any growth requirements specific to the strain. Some workers prefer to use yeast complete broth diluted to one-fifth strength (Sharp & Parry, 1981; Zimmermann & Scheel, 1981) rather than complete medium to minimise scavenging of the test compound by components of the growth medium. If required, the minimal medium can be buffered using a final concentration of 100 mM phosphate (Zimmermann, Mayer & Parry, 1982). The yeast culture should be incubated in a suitable (e.g. conical) flask at 28 °C on an orbital shaker until the cells are growing exponentially. This usually takes about 6 h but will vary from strain to strain. The cell titre and the percentage of cells with small buds (less than one-third the size of the parental cell) should then be determined using a haemocytometer. Bud emergence has been shown to coincide with the onset of DNA replication (Hartwell, 1974). In an exponentially growing cell culture under optimal conditions, around 20% of the cells should have small buds. The cell titre should be adjusted as required by diluting with prewarmed minimal broth or allowing further growth. The number of cells used at the start of treatment will depend on the generation time of the particular strain and the length of treatment. The essential criterion is that, during treatment, the medium should not become exhausted such that the cells enter stationary phase, as this can favour the selection of prototrophic cells.

Aliquots of the bulk yeast culture should be dispensed into the treatment vessels and mixed immediately with the test agent and the S9-mix if used. The cells should have reasonable aeration during treatment so it is necessary to provide a relatively large air space above the treatment mix. If small volumes (for example, 2 ml) are used, 30 ml universal bottles are adequate. Some workers prefer to use large volumes and treat in conical flasks. The individual bottles should then be incubated at 28–30 °C with shaking. For treatment in the presence of S9 an initial incubation period (up to 2 h) at 37 °C is recommended (see Section 2.3.9.1). Orbital shakers are preferable to horizontal shaking water baths, as the cells tend to settle out of suspension with the latter. With many mutagenic chemicals, good dose–response curves can be obtained with short treatment times; however, with compounds of unknown activity an overnight exposure of 16 or 18 h is recommended. Longer treatment times than this increase the possibility of sporulation. With suspect or known photosensitive chemicals, treatment should be carried out both in the light and in the dark to determine whether this affects genetic activity (Fahrig, 1976; Callen & Larson, 1978).

After the prescribed period, treatment should be terminated by successive washings with ice-cold saline. For experiments with known alkylating agents, the cells can be washed with cold 10% sodium thiosulphate to inactivate the test compound (Parry & Parry, 1984). The cells should then be resuspended in saline at a cell titre suitable for plating (usually about $1-2 \times 10^7$ cells per ml). At this stage, the cells should be examined microscopically and checked for the presence of asci to ensure that sporulation has not been induced. The cells should be plated as soon as possible after cessation of treatment (same day) and kept on ice or in a refrigerator until this time. Before plating, the cell suspension should be vigorously agitated using a vortex mixer to attempt to break up clusters. This can be checked microscopically. Some workers briefly sonicate the cell suspensions for this purpose. Small volumes (usually 100 μl) of undiluted suspension should be pipetted onto the centre of the selective plates and spread evenly over the surface with a glass rod. The glass rod can be sterilised by flaming in alcohol, but care should be taken to cool the rod on the surface of the plate before contact with the cells. A minimum of three plates of each type should be used for each treatment. The number of cells plated onto the selective plates should be such that a reliable count is obtained on the control plates (preferably not less than 20) for calculating the spontaneous frequency. With most heteroallelic markers, this usually requires about 1×10^6 cells per plate. To assess survival, the cells should be diluted in isotonic saline and plated onto complete medium to give ideally between 100 and 200 colonies per plate. It is usually advisable to plate out at several different dilutions to ensure that satisfactory counts are obtained if the test compound is toxic to the yeast cells.

The plates are then incubated at 28–30 °C in the dark. Survival plates can usually be scored after 2–3 days and the selective plates after about 5 days, although this will depend on the strain and genetic markers being used. Also some chemicals may retard cell growth and slow down colony formation. Automatic colony counters can give rise to problems when counting yeast, as colonies may be large and frequently touching, particularly on complete plates; colonies may also be very variable in size on selective plates. The number of colonies on the selective and complete plates should be recorded and the conversion frequency with the different treatments calculated. If the strain showed problems of clustering, the results should be expressed as convertants per colony-forming unit.

Some workers have used protocols in which exponentially growing cells are resuspended and treated in buffer (Callen & Philpott, 1977; Callen, Wolf & Philpot, 1980; Parry, 1982; Callen, 1981). Such cells are usually capable of at least one subsequent cell division in the buffer. This method prevents scavenging effects by components of the growth medium and the problems of low pH with growing cultures. However, the method is only suitable for short treatment times and is not recommended for initial screening.

(b)   *Treatment of stationary phase cells*

In view of the problems in treating growing cells, mutagenic chemicals often give better dose–response curves with stationary phase cultures. Cells should be grown to the end of log phase in liquid medium or on agar plates. The time this takes will vary from strain to strain and should be determined in each laboratory. Cells grown in liquid medium should be washed free of medium by repeated centrifugation and resuspended in buffer of the required pH. There are circumstances at which the tolerance of yeast to pH values from 3 to 9 may be utilised (Zetterberg, 1979); however, for general screening purposes we recommend that assays be performed at pH7. Cells grown on plates can be scraped off with a sterile spatula and resuspended directly in buffer. The cell titre and percentage of cells with small buds should be determined using a haemocytometer. In stationary phase cultures less than 5% of cells should have small buds. The cell titre should be adjusted to about 2×10^7 cells per ml as is required for most strains. Aliquots of this suspension should then be dispensed into the treatment bottles and treatment and plating carried out as described for growing cells. Overnight exposures of 16 or 18 h are again recommended for initial experiments. The remainder of the procedure is as discussed in (a).

2.3.3.2   *Mitotic crossing-over*

Unambiguous demonstration of mitotic crossing-over requires the identification of both reciprocal products of recombination. This can be achieved in strains D5 (Zimmermann, 1973b) and D7 (Zimmermann, 1975) using the *ade*2–40/*ade*–119 system. Treated cells should be plated at about 200 cells per plate onto yeast complete plates containing only 5 mg per litre adenine and incubated at 28–30 °C for 6–8 days. A further incubation period at 4 °C aids formation of the red pigment in the colonies. The plates should then be scored for total colony count and for red and pink whole colonies, twin colonies and sectors. The frequency of the different types should be recorded separately. An increase in the frequency of pink/red twin colonies is definitive evidence of mitotic reciprocal crossing-over. In practice, these twin colonies are only obtained if stationary phase cells are treated, since in growing cultures the two products of recombination will separate on cell division and give rise to independent colonies. The method is not suitable for routine use because of the large number of colonies that have to be screened.

Many of the strains used for the detection of other genetic events possess additional markers which can be used to score mitotic crossing-over between the gene and the centromere. Examples are the induction of red *ade2* colonies in JD1 and cycloheximide-resistant colonies in D6. These can be detected quite easily with JD1 by scoring the frequency of red colonies on yeast complete plates (with low adenine) and with D6 by plating onto yeast complete plates containing 2 mg per litre cycloheximide. Although these are not recommended as test systems in themselves, an increase in the frequency of these events would add weight to positive findings with other genetic markers in the strain.

2.3.3.3 *Intrachromosomal recombination*

As discussed in Section 2.2.2, a yeast strain RS112 has recently been developed containing a system to select for intrachromosomal recombination (Schiestl *et al.*, 1988).

It should be noted that when using strain RS112 to measure intra-chromosomal deletion events the culture should be grown in liquid minimal media containing all the strain's requirements, except for leucine, for 24 hours before use (Schiestl *et al.*, 1989). This ensures that the culture contains a low background of cells which have lost the plasmid pBR322 and has a spontaneous frequency of approximately 1 histidine revertant per 10^4 viable cells.

We cannot recommend this strain for general use, and reserve detailed discussion pending further validation studies.

2.3.3.4 *Gene mutation*

(*a*)   *Reverse mutation systems*

The protocols used for measuring reverse mutation at auxotrophic loci are essentially the same as for mitotic gene conversion, except that a higher number of cells has to be plated onto the selective plates. For commonly used base-pair substitution loci, usually about $1-2 \times 10^7$ cells per plate are required, but this will depend on the individual strain and marker. The number of cells plated should be sufficient to produce a reliable colony count on the control plates. With the frameshift auxotrophic markers available in yeast, this can prove difficult since the spontaneous reversion frequency is very low. At least 1×10^8 cells per plate are required to give any sort of count on the control plates. It is difficult to work with cell suspensions of more than about 2×10^8 cells per ml, so to achieve the number of cells required to detect reversion by frameshift, large volumes of culture at a lower cell titre (1×10^8 cells per ml) can be treated. These can then be concentrated to 5×10^8 cells per ml after washing and 200 μl applied to the selective plates. With this number of cells, agar overlay techniques can give more consistent results than spreading the cells on the surface of the plates. A sample can be removed before addition of the molten salt agar for assessing cell survival. Plating heavy suspensions of yeast cells can sometimes give problems of medium depletion or cryptic feeding (Zimmermann, 1975)

(b)   *Forward mutation systems*

(i)   *Ade2* system

Treatment protocols are as described for mitotic gene conversion. Treated cells should be washed free of chemical and plated onto yeast complete plates containing 5 mg per litre adenine (Zimmermann, 1975) with the aim of yielding about 200 colonies per plate. These should be incubated for 2–3 days at 30 °C for the colonies to grow up. A further incubation period at 4 °C (for about 2 days) aids formation of the red colour in colonies. The plates should then be scored for total colony count to assess cell survival and for white colonies or sectors to assess forward mutations in the adenine loci which precede the *ade2* block. A minimum of 20 000 colonies per treatment (i.e. about 100 plates) should be scored for compounds which show no activity (Brusick, 1980). Some workers prefer to score for white colonies by plating out at higher cell densities (about 1000 cells per plate) and using a low power microscope to examine the plates. Owing to the large number of colonies that have to be scored, the method is very labour intensive and consequently has not been used to screen large numbers of compounds.

However, the assay is scientifically robust and may have an application in special cases where equivocal results are obtained in other systems. One possible pitfall with the method is that formation of the red colour in respiratory-deficient colonies is poor and such colonies may be misclassified by inexperienced workers (Brusick & Andrews, 1974).

(ii)   Resistance to toxic agents

With these systems, there is a necessity to provide a period of post-treatment growth under non-selective conditions to allow for phenotypic lag. For example, in the canavanine resistance system, if cells are plated directly onto canavanine medium, copies of the normal arginine permease enzyme will still exist even in mutant cells. Consequently, until there has been time for induced mutations to be expressed, even mutated cells will be sensitive to the lethal effects of canavanine. Lemontt (1977) found that a post-treatment expression time of 11 h in yeast complete growth medium gave maximum recovery of mutants. However, from a practical aspect, an overnight growth period is often used.

2.3.3.5 *Mitotic aneuploidy*

Since the production of aneuploid cells is generally a function of inaccurate cell division, the treatment of actively dividing cells is essential for this endpoint. However, allowing too much growth can also give rise to problems since aneuploid cells, once induced, can be selected against in cultures comprising predominantly euploid cells. In order to reduce growth during the treatment period some workers have advocated using two-fifths strength yeast complete medium (Parry, Sharp & Parry, 1979; Parry & Sharp, 1981; Albertini *et al.*, 1985). For strains D6 and D61.M most published protocols involve treating growing cultures overnight (16–18 h), after which the compound is removed by washing in ice-cold saline and, if necessary, the cell titre readjusted to around 4–6×10^7 cells per ml. Aneuploid colonies are detected by plating 100 µl of this suspension onto yeast complete plates containing 1.5–2 mg per litre cycloheximide and only 5 mg per litre adenine. Toxicity is assessed by diluting and plating onto yeast complete plates without cycloheximide and counting the total number of colonies after 3–4 days' growth. The cycloheximide plates should be scored for small white colonies after 6 (D61.M) or 10 (D6) days' growth. The use of a low power microscope can assist in this process. As discussed earlier, to provide definitive proof of aneuploidy it is essential to demonstrate simultaneous expression of the nutritional marker(s) present on chromosome VII (leu for D61.M; leu, met or trp for D6). This can be achieved by carefully picking off suspected aneuploid colonies, streaking into yeast complete plates, growing overnight and then replica plating onto yeast minimal medium supplemented with all the growth requirements except the marker being investigated, e.g. leucine. Zimmermann *et al.* (1984*a*, 1985*a*, 1986) have described a protocol modification which resulted in a significantly higher yield of aneuploid colonies with a series of aprotic solvents, e.g. acetone, acetonitrile. This involves treating growing cells for 4 h at 30 °C, then placing the cultures in an ice bath for 16 h, and finally allowing another 4 h growth at 30 °C. The period at 0 °C causes tubulin to depolymerise and this appears to aid the detection of aneugens that act via interference with tubulin assembly (Zimmermann *et al.*, 1985*a*, *b*). This modification has little effect on the results obtained with aneugens that work by a different mechanism, and whether it should be used as part of a primary screen probably depends on the nature of the compounds being investigated.

2.3.3.6   Petite induction

The ultimate criterion for scoring petite mutants is their inability to grow on non-fermentable carbon sources, such as glycerol. To assess the frequency of petites, the total number of viable cells and the number of petites must be established. This can be achieved by plating cells onto yeast complete medium, allowing the colonies to grow up and then replica plating onto glycerol plates. This technique, however, does not always give clear results. A more suitable method for identifying petite colonies has been developed by Ogur, John & Nagai (1957), based on the inability of petite cells to metabolise 2,3,5-triphenyltetrazolium chloride.

The induction of petite mutations by chemical agents appears to be very strain specific (Egilsson, Evans & Wilkie, 1979; Patel & Wilkie, 1982; Ferguson, 1984). For screening of novel compounds Ferguson (1984) has recommended using three strains, ise 1-2, 5178B and D5. It has been shown that, for some compounds, treatment of growing cells gives optimal petite induction, but for others, treating stationary phase cells in isotonic saline gives a better response (Iwamoto *et al.*, 1986; Ferguson & Turner, 1988). Consequently, when screening novel compounds both conditions should be employed, with a treatment period of around 16–24 h. Ferguson (1984) has described a cost-effective method of exposure in which cells are treated with a range of concentrations of test agent in microtitre trays.

Treated cells should be plated onto yeast complete medium containing 1% glucose. After 2–3 days' growth, the colonies should be counted and the counts recorded on the individual plates. The plates should then be carefully overlaid with molten (50 °C) soft agar buffered at pH 7.0 and containing 1 mg per ml of triphenyltetrazolium. The tetrazolium solution should be added to the molten agar immediately before overlaying, as autoclaving in the presence of agar reduces the tetrazolium. The plates should be left for 2–3 h on the bench before scoring. Normal 'grande' colonies can rapidly metabolise triphenyltetrazolium to an intermediate which turns the colonies red in colour. Petite cells are unable to carry out this conversion, or at least do so very slowly, and remain white. The total cell count on the complete plates can be used to estimate toxicity and the percentage of petite colonies at each treatment calculated. The more colonies scored, the more reliable the estimation of petite frequency. The method does seem to have a certain amount of inherent variability and only clear dose-related increases should be considered as a positive effect.

The relevance of mitochondrial mutations to carcinogenic or mutagenic hazard is uncertain. While many tumour cells have been shown to possess functionally defective mitochondria, it is far from clear whether this is one of the causative steps in the transformation process or a consequential event (Wilkie *et al.*, 1983; Shay & Werbin, 1987). At present, we would not recommend that an assay for petite induction be considered as a basic screening test for genotoxic activity. However, the assay may have other uses, for example, exploring the potential of the mitochondria as a target for chemotherapy (Ferguson & Turner, 1988; Baguley, Turner & Ferguson, 1990).

2.3.4 Phenotypic lag

With bacterial mutation systems based on the reversion of auxotrophic strains, it is customary to provide the cells with a trace amount of the growth requirement to allow for expression of induced mutations. With comparable assays for mitotic gene conversion, however, this is not essential since gene conversion can occur in G1 cells (Fabre, 1978) and there is no requirement for post-treatment DNA replication or growth. In fact, even with yeast reverse mutation systems, there is no need to include trace supplement in the selective plates, as it appears that the intracellular metabolite pools are sufficient to allow phenotypic expression of any induced mutations. The only yeast assay with which there appears to be a problem of phenotypic lag is the forward mutation system based on resistance to toxic agents, e.g. canavanine, discussed previously.

2.3.5 Problems of sporulation with diploid cultures

As mentioned earlier, uncontrolled sporulation during treatment with chemical agents can give rise to very misleading results. After treatment, cell populations should therefore be visually screened for the presence of asci to check that sporulation has not occurred. This method is not entirely satisfactory since very low frequencies of sporulation, which may go undetected, could still be sufficient to result in a false positive assessment. To complement visual screening, some strains carry additional colony-colour markers which can be useful in assessing whether sporulation has occurred. For example, if sporulation is induced in a strain heterozygous for *ade*2-40, 50% of the resulting haploids will be red in colour. The presence of unusually high numbers of red colonies on the yeast complete plates, therefore, indicates that sporulation may have occurred. Red colonies can also be generated in such strains by mitotic reciprocal crossing-over. These colonies will be diploids which are homoallelic at the *ade*2-40 locus. Picking off a few red colonies and checking their ploidy can differentiate between these two events.

Some groups have overcome the problem of uncontrolled sporulation by using petite isolates which are unable to sporulate. With certain mutagenic compounds these petite isolates appear to be more sensitive than the original 'grande' strains (Zimmermann, 1969; Mayer, Hybner & Brusick, 1976;

Siebert, Bayer & Marquardt, 1979; Wilcox, 1984). However, if such strains are used, the possibility that petite cells may metabolise foreign compounds in different ways to 'grande' cells must be borne in mind. Yeast strains have been constructed with specific blocks in the sporulation process, but which are normal in terms of respiratory competence, such as strain D7-114 (Mehta & von Borstel, 1985).

2.3.6   Induction versus selection

With all yeast assays based on selective systems, the possibility that positive results could be due to selection of pre-existing mutants rather than induced genetic events must always be considered. Selection can occur through differential killing of non-revertant cells or, with protocols using growing cells, if conditions are created which favour the growth of pre-existing mutants rather than the normal unmutated cells. With stationary phase protocols, if an absolute increase in revertant colonies per plate is observed on the selective medium, this can be assumed to be due to an induced genetic effect and there is no need to check for selection. However, if there is no increase in revertant colonies per plate, but when toxicity is taken into account a calculated increase in revertants per surviving cell is obtained, it would be prudent to demonstrate that selection has not occurred. This can be achieved by conducting reconstruction experiments which compare the toxicity of the chemical in normal cells and in cells derived from a revertant clone. If the toxicity of the compound in normal and revertant cells is identical, then selective effects by differential killing can be ruled out. For experiments with growing cells, selection can be checked by comparing the growth rates of normal and revertant cells in the presence of the test agent.

2.3.7   Dose selection and controls
2.3.7.1   *Dose selection*

The basic experimental design with yeast mutagenicity assays is very similar to that recommended for *in vitro* bacterial tests. Compounds should be tested at four or five different dose levels, which should be spaced on a geometric scale at two- to three-fold concentration intervals. Ideally, the highest dose used should produce a significant reduction in survival (say to 10% viability) and the lower doses should show no toxicity. Concentrations which reduce survival to less than 10% should not be used routinely (Zimmermann, 1975). If a sharp decrease in survival between consecutive dose levels is obtained, a repeat assay may be necessary using closer spaced doses around the toxic level. With test compounds which do not produce toxicity, the highest concentration can be selected on the basis of just exceeding maximum solubility; there is little point in testing beyond this concentration. For very soluble, non-toxic compounds, the criteria for selecting the top dose level are more difficult. However, if a chemical does not induce genetic effects at a concentration of 5 mg per ml, it is unlikely that it will do so at higher doses. Special cases may have to be made with very reactive or unstable compounds. Positive results, obtained only at very high dose levels, may be due to the presence of mutagenic impurities in the test chemical.

When screening for mitotic aneuploidy, the effective concentration range can be very narrow (see Zimmermann *et al.*, 1985*b*; Piegorsch *et al.*, 1989); for example, with spindle inhibitors, too little compound can have no effect, whereas too much can totally block cell division.

2.3.7.2 Controls

(*a*)   Negative controls

All experiments should include a solvent control which should be added at the highest level (vol/vol) used with the test compound. Solvents which have been widely used with yeast assays include water, dimethyl-sulphoxide (DMSO), acetone and ethanol. Each laboratory should demonstrate that the solvents it employs do not induce genetic effects or produce toxicity at the levels used. DMSO has been reported to induce mitotic gene conversion in yeast (Callen & Philpot, 1977) if used at high concentration (above 1 M). Up to 5% DMSO, however, does not induce detectable gene conversion or produce toxicity. Mayer and Goin (1987) have reported that relatively low levels of DMSO (i.e. below 5% v/v) can reduce the yield of aneuploid cells after treatment with nocodazole or ethyl acetate, therefore it would be prudent to avoid this solvent, if possible, when screening for chromosome loss. Also, acetone has been reported to induce chromosome loss in D61.M at concentrations between 5 and 10% v/v (Zimmermann *et al.*, 1984*b*, 1985*a*).

It is important that the spontaneous mutation frequency of the genetic markers being employed should be monitored in each experiment and, if this falls outside the usual range, the assay should usually be rejected. This is particularly important with assays for mitotic gene conversion, since over-selection of heteroallelic markers can lead to the establishment of the homoallelic state (by mitotic crossing-over). If this occurs, reversion can only be achieved by back mutation and not mitotic gene conversion. The spontaneous reversion frequency will therefore be much lower and the marker may become mutagen specific, for example, responding to only base pair substitution mutagens. Increases in the spontaneous frequency may indicate a high level of pre-existing revertants in the culture which may mask weak induced effects. Unusually high control levels with diploid strains may also indicate that sporulation has occurred.

(*b*)   *Positive controls*

The correct use of positive control chemicals has been discussed in general in Chapter 1. A range of direct and indirect-acting positive control chemicals suitable for use in yeast genotoxicity assays is given in Table 2.1.

2.3.8   Maintenance of stock cultures

Yeast cultures can be maintained on yeast complete plates or slopes at 4 °C for up to one year. Although this gives satisfactory results with some strains, it is not advisable to rely totally on this method as some strains may sporulate under these conditions. Permanent stock cultures can be prepared by lyophilisation or by absorbing onto silica gel in the cold (Zimmermann, 1973*a*).

Alternatively, long-term storage may be accomplished by freeze drying cultures that have been suspended in double strength skimmed milk, or half strength fresh growth medium containing 12% sucrose. To recover fungi from freeze-dried specimens, it is recommended that 0.3–0.4 ml of sterile water is aseptically added to the culture, mixed well and soaked for at least 30 minutes before transferring the total mixture to a test-tube of the appropriate growth medium (5–6 ml). The last few drops of this suspension may also be transferred to an agar plate.

It is also possible to store cultures over liquid nitrogen or at −70 °C in a deep freeze; 10% glycerol or dimethyl sulphoxide should be added to the medium as a cryptoprotective agent and it is recommended that the cells be frozen down slowly at a rate of about 1 °C per minute. Strains of *S. cerevisiae* have been flash frozen in liquid nitrogen with no adverse effects even after glycerol concentrations reached 50% in the medium. Cells remain viable under these conditions for periods of several years. On recovery of strains from storage, it is strongly recommended that all essential genetic markers should be checked before the strain is used for testing. Zimmermann (1975) recommends that, for each experiment, replicate cultures are grown from individual clones and stored at 4 °C whilst the spontaneous reversion level in each culture is determined. A culture which gives a normal spontaneous level can then be used for the full experiment. With certain strains, such as *ade*2 mutants this procedure may be advisable, but this is usually unnecessary if cultures are properly maintained.

2.3.9   Activation systems

2.3.9.1   *Exogenous activation system*

Bioactivation is a pre-requisite for the detection of many carcinogens as mutagens. Such reactions are usually catalysed by Phase I oxidative enzymes, e.g. cytochrome P450. Metabolic activation of promutagens *in vitro*

Table 2.1. *Some examples of chemicals suitable for use as positive controls in yeast assays*

Genetic endpoint	Chemical
Mitotic gene conversion and nuclear gene mutation	*Direct acting* ethylmethane sulphonate, methylmethane sulphonate, 4-nitroquinoline oxide, nitrous acid, hycanthone
	Indirect acting 2-acetylaminofluorene, 2-aminofluorene, sterigmatocystin, cyclophosphamide
Cytoplasmic petite mutation	*Direct acting* ethidium bromide acriflavine
	Indirect acting benzidine
Mitotic chromosome aneuploidy	*Direct acting* benomyl sodium deoxycholate
	Indirect acting cyclophosphamide

is generally achieved by the addition of mammalian microsomal monooxygenases usually in the form of the 9000G supernatant fraction (S9) from rodent liver (Ames *et al.*, 1975). The most common S9 mix used is that from Aroclor-induced rat liver, although some groups have successfully used phenobarbitone/β-naphthoflavone-induced liver (Paolini *et al.*, 1990).

Variations in the proportions of cofactors and protein levels differ between laboratories (see, for example, Loprieno, 1981; Sharp & Parry, 1981), although most laboratories use an S9 mix based on the method of Ames *et al.* (1975).

A widely accepted method for general screening in yeast is to add S9 mix to the yeast culture and test substance in liquid in a treat-and-plate method. Parry and Parry (1984) recommended a protocol using 50 μl–150 μl of S9-mix added to 1 ml yeast cells (stationary or logarithmic phase) and 100 μl test compound in a suitable solvent, the whole being made up to a final volume of 2 ml with phosphate buffer pH 7.0 and incubated at 37 °C for 2 h without shaking and then at 28 °C for 16 h on an orbital shaker.

Probably the most significant difference in the use of liver homogenates between the Ames test and yeast assays is that the latter involve liquid treatments. In such liquid assays, the 'life-time' of S9 mix is relatively short.

Although yeasts grow optimally at around 30 °C, for treatments in the presence of S9 mix, an initial incubation period at 37 °C is recommended as mammalian enzymes function better at this temperature; there is little point extending this 37 °C incubation period beyond 2 h as the enzymes will no longer be active after this time (Leadbeater & Davis, 1964).

2.3.9.2 *Endogenous activation system*

A potential advantage of the use of yeasts is that, unlike bacteria, they possess an electron transfer (oxidative) system analogous to that found in mammals. The presence of cytochrome P450 in yeast was first demonstrated by Lindenmayer and Smith (1964). Since then, various other components of the electron transport system have also been identified. The molecular cloning of various genes of the *S. cerevisiae* system has been reported. A cytochrome P450 has been cloned (Kalb *et al.*, 1986) and analysis of the gene sequence and phenotype of the disrupted mutants has identified the cyt P450 as being the sterol C14 demethylase enzyme. From studies on mutant strains and from protein purification studies, this enzyme appears to be the predominant cyt P450 form present during semi-anaerobic growth (Kalb *et al.*, 1986; Yoshida & Aoyama, 1984; Stansfield, Cliffe & Kelly, 1991) and has been assigned to a separate group within the superfamily, P450LIAI (Nebert *et al.*, 1987) or CYP51 (Nebert *et al.*, 1991). More recently, a second putative yeast cyt P450 involved in spore wall maturation has been cloned (Briza *et al.*, 1990). It has low (only 12%) homology with the P450LIAI gene. The yeast cyt P450 reductase has also been cloned (Yabusaki, Murakami & Ohkawa, 1988) and its functional domains have been found to closely resemble those of its mammalian counterparts.

The cellular content of cyt P450LIAI has been shown to vary over a wide range depending on the growth conditions, depression or induction and the stage of the life-cycle (Wiseman, Lim & McCloud, 1975*a*). The concentration of P450LIAI in anaerobically grown cells falls rapidly upon aeration and also at late stages of the cell cycle if grown on lower glucose concentrations (1% w/v). If higher glucose concentrations (up to 20% w/v) in the growth medium are used, the concentration of cyt P450LIAI remains higher for a longer period of the yeast growth phase (Blatiak, Gondal & Wiseman, 1980). Glucose depletion leads to depression of cyt P450LIAI. Yeast grown under conditions of high glucose have shown the ability to metabolise biphenyl by hydroxy-lation to the 4-hydroxylate derivative (Wiseman, Gondal & Sims, 1975*b*) and also to show demethylase activity when treated with N-ethyl morphine and aminopyrine (Wiseman, Jay & Gondal, 1975*c*).

Callen & Philpot (1977) demonstrated that growth of *S. cerevisiae* in medium with 2% w/v glucose concentration led to increased cyt P450 levels and, under these conditions, the strains D4 and D5 were capable of metabolic activation of certain chemicals to genotoxic species. This protocol did not optimise the level of cyt P450 present over long treatment times. However, an assay system based on transferring cells grown in low glucose (0.5% w/v) to high (20% w/v) glucose containing medium has been shown to produce increased levels of cyt P450 and a slower rate of disappearance than under aerobic conditions (Kelly & Parry, 1983). This is of particular importance when treatment times take up to 18 h. Cells grown from an initial inoculum of 1×10^3 cells per ml to 1×10^7 cells per ml in 0.5% (w/v) glucose complete medium are resuspended in 20% (w/v) glucose complete medium. Treatment of 2 ml aliquots with the test chemical follow the same treat-and-plate regime described in Section 2.3.3.1. A modification of this protocol (Parry and Eckardt, 1985*a*, *b*) involves delaying the treatment of cells until 4 h or 6 h after transferring to 20% glucose medium, so that cyt P450 levels are already elevated at the time of adding the test compound (Parry & Parry, 1984).

Hrelia *et al.* (1987) have reported that nitro-reductive enzymes are also inducible under the same high glucose (20% w/v) medium conditions and that nitroimidazo (2,1-β) thiazoles were genetically active in strain D7 when tested in growing cells as opposed to stationary phase cells.

Using protocols which give elevated levels of cyt P450 in growing cells it has been demonstrated that the yeast cyt P450 is able to metabolise a number of compounds to genotoxic species (Kelly & Parry, 1983; del Carratore *et al.*, 1983; Niggli *et al.*, 1986; Niggli, Friederich & Würgler, 1988; Koch, Schlegelmilch & Wolf, 1988). However, not all compounds are substrates for the yeast enzyme (Jagannath *et al.*, 1985; Koch, Schlegelmilch & Wolf, 1988). Thus, assays with and without S9 should always be used for general screening purposes.

The narrow substrate specificity of the yeast monooxygenase system may be overcome in the future by the cloning and overexpression of different mammalian cyt P450s in yeast (Oeda, Sakaki & Ohkawa, 1985; Imai, 1988; Black *et al.*, 1989; Yasumori *et al.*, 1989; Eugster *et al.*, 1990; Ching *et al.*, 1991). Heterologous cyt P450 expression in yeast cells involves self-replicating plasmids containing a selectable marker and the P450 cDNA coding sequence inserted between a yeast transcription promoter and a terminator sequence. More usually, expression vectors utilising strong constitutive yeast promoters such as the PGK (phosphoglycerate kinase) and ADH (alcohol dehydrogenase) are used, although inducible promoters such as different GAL (galactose) and PHO5 (phosphase) have also been tried.

The expressed cyt P450s have been shown to couple to the yeast reductase and be functional. It is thought that simultaneous overexpression of cyt b_5 and cyt P450 reductase is necessary to obtain optimal activity of foreign P450s in yeast. Targeted integration of the human cyt b_5 and the P450 reductase genes into the yeast genome, under the control of inducible promoters, has allowed the expression levels of these associated enzymes to be controlled independently of the heterologous P450 level (Urban, Cullin & Pompon, 1990). Such a yeast strain has been called 'humanised' and this approach is also being extended to encompass phase II enzymes, e.g. human epoxide hydrolase (Eugster *et al.*, 1988; Urban *et al.*, 1990). The use of growing cells expressing functional human microsomal enzymes or the use of yeast microsomes prepared from them offer the opportunity to investigate the metabolism of mutagens/carcinogens by human cytochrome P450 enzymes.

2.4   ANALYSIS OF DATA

Because there are no commonly used experimental designs for yeast, there have been few attempts to devise suitable statistical analyses for the data. Therefore it is inevitable that the approaches used will be derived from those applied to the more common genotoxicity assays.

General aspects of genotoxicity data analyses have been reviewed in recent literature (Mitchell, 1987; Lovell, 1989). Agar plate assays and fluctuation tests are uncommon in yeast. There are comprehensive reviews of statistical analyses for these methodologies with bacterial assays (Mahon *et al.*, 1989; Robinson *et al.*, 1989) which are directly applicable to yeast systems. Thus we shall not discuss these methods further.

Statistical analyses for mammalian 'treat and plate' assays have also been reviewed in relation to mammalian cell mutagenicity assays (Arlett *et al.*, 1989). However, there are many cases where the methodology cannot be directly applied to yeast experiments because test design and spontaneous frequencies are very different and the aim of the reviewers (Arlett *et al.*, 1989) was to provide an analysis for a very specific test system and design.

2.4.1   Theoretical and practical limitations for statistical methodology

On theoretical considerations, the problem is finding a statistical analysis for approximately normal distributions of unequal and unstable variance. Several possible solutions suggest themselves; transformation of data followed by parametric analysis (Bartlett, 1947; Box & Cox, 1964), use of weighted variances followed by parametric analyses (Arlett *et al.*, 1989), use of the Bayesian solution to the Behrens–Fisher problem (Box & Tiao, 1973) and a variety of non-parametric analyses based on the Wilcoxon statistic U (e.g. Mann–Whitney U test), normal scores (e.g. Terry–Hoeffding test) and maximum deviation (e.g. Kolmogorov–Smirnov two-sample test) (Bradley, 1968; Campbell, 1974*a*).

The treatment flask is the unit of statistical analysis because there is usually significant flask-to-flask non-statistical variation and also a significant amount of test variance arises at inoculation. Practically, the number of flasks used in any one test is severely limited. There are technical constraints on the number that can be managed and theoretical limits on the maximum size of combined inoculum due to insensitivity. Thus it is difficult to assay the required number of concentration levels (four or five) and also build sufficient replication into one test to either permit non-parametric analysis, or to calculate test variance accurately from concurrent data. The latter severely limits the reliability of most of the applicable parametric analyses. An added complication is the lack of easily available transformations (Box & Cox, 1964) for the complex type of variance (with many components) in data from 'treat and plate' assays. Thus the requirement for constant (stable) variance is difficult to meet. However, either square root or log transformation (Bartlett, 1947) would probably assist where the treated and control means were not 'too different' (i.e. where statistics are really needed).

2.4.2 Some suggested solutions and their problems

The solution recommended by Arlett *et al.* (1989) was to apply ANOVA and linear regression analysis using weighted variance to overcome the lack of a suitable transformation. Two methods of weighting were suggested; one using variance calculated from concurrent data which was acknowledged to be very inaccurate and a second using variance assumed to be Poisson. Some of the assumptions and manipulations in this methodology seem to us of questionable applicability but, overall, offer a reasonable, if complicated, parametric solution for appropriate study designs.

A second suggestion was to make use of the historical data base (Arlett *et al.*, 1989) and a method of doing this has been suggested (Mitchell *et al.*, 1990). The latter method of using control ratios is better than previously used variance coefficients based on historical data (Mitchell & Gilbert, 1984) as no assumption of normality or constant variance is made. The basic objection to the use of historical data is that there will always be some degree of test-to-test variation (Murphy, Caspary & Margolin, 1988). Also there are problems when survival falls, and data have to be scaled to give mutation frequencies.

An older method was to use chi-squared analysis or its parametric binomial-based equivalent (Kastenbaum & Bowman, 1970). This approach has fallen out of favour because it took no account of flask to flask variation and data from different flasks were treated as homogeneous which they clearly are not. However, declining survival is no problem in chi-squared analysis. Overall, we consider chi-squared analysis to be of dubious validity but it may be used provided that a likely over-estimate of significance is acknowledged.

Finally, where the negative control and various treatment levels are compared pairwise a correction is needed for overall test significance. Various approaches are possible (Mitchell, 1987) but where a combined analysis (e.g. ANOVA) is inappropriate a Bonferroni correction (Abt, 1981) is acceptable.

However, the whole issue of methodology for protection against type I (α) errors with multiple comparisons is a subject of controversy amongst statisticians and there are no wholly satisfactory solutions.

Assays must now include an independent repeat experiment for regulatory purposes. It seems unnecessary that the same design is used for both tests. Thus we suggest that the first test should be a screening test over several (four or five) concentrations. Concentration–response trends could then be statistically analysed by a method based on Kendall's coefficient of rank correlation (Campbell, 1974*b*) or by the Cochran–Armitage linear trend test (Snedecor & Cochran, 1967).

Pairwise comparisons between the negative control and treatments could be made by chi-squared analysis (acknowledging a possible over-estimate of significance) combined with a Bonferroni correction for test significance. The results could be checked against historical data (Mitchell *et al.*, 1990). Alternatively, a Dunnett's test on log or square root transformed data would probably yield a more reliable estimate of the significance of any one test concentration provided there was sufficient replication in the test. It should be noted that replication means identical tests run in parallel (at the same time) and should not be confused with repeat tests which are always performed on separate occasions and often do not use the same test design. The design of the repeat test should be governed by observations in the first (initial) assay, and is used to resolve any problems therein.

Finally, it is often useful to consult a statistician prior to embarking on a set of experiments because individual designs can vary considerably. Therefore, the suggestions in this section may be neither optimal nor, in some cases, applicable. However, generally, they will provide a useful, initial framework.

2.5   CONCLUSION

The yeast assays described here provide a convenient set of protocols for evaluating the genotoxicity of environmental chemicals in simple eukaryotic cells. Within a single species a wide range of genetic endpoints may be studied in the appropriate strains with relatively minor variations in protocols. For general screening purposes, it is our view that the most convenient yeast assay is that for the induction of mitotic gene conversion using a well validated strain and protocol. The other endpoints discussed may be used to complement this test if they are of particular interest and if there is other information available to indicate that the test compound might be effective at inducing the particular endpoint.

For general screening purposes using mitotic gene conversion as the endpoint, we recommend that the initial test should be in log-phase cultures. If this test proves clearly negative, then a similar stationary phase test should be carried out. Negative data from two such tests are sufficient to define a negative result. Any equivocal or weakly positive result could be retested at one or more appropriate concentrations used with negative control and treated samples replicated four or five times. The concentration(s) for this confirmatory test would be based on the results from the first screening tests. The test could then be analysed by any of the methods suggested at the beginning of Section 2.4.1. We have a marginal preference for the non-parametric approach because the assumption of normality is theoretical. In practice, biological distributions are often skewed. Any definite positive result in a first assay should be further investigated to establish a dose (concentration)–response curve.

The following factors should be carefully considered in evaluating the results of a yeast assay:

1. The spontaneous frequency of the marker being used must be within the usual range for the testing laboratory.
2. The induced mutation/conversion, etc. frequency with the positive control should be within the usual range for the testing laboratory.
3. The activity of the S9 fraction and endogenous potential should be demonstrated by a suitable positive control.
4. The compound should be tested over a suitable concentration range and, preferably, at a minimum of four to five dose levels.
5. For compounds showing no activity, assays should be carried out using both growing and stationary phase cells.
6. Overnight exposure to the test chemical should be used in at least one assay.
7. Where appropriate, checks for artefacts due to sporulation or selection should be carried out.

In addition to their role in general screening, yeast assays may be selected to fill specific niches in comprehensive test programmes. For example, the yeast aneuploidy assays and the induction of mitochondrial mutations are almost unique in determining the potential of chemicals to induce such endpoints in organisms that can be handled by conventional microbiological techniques.

Also, the use of yeast in molecular biology has led to the integration of human cytochrome P450 genes, and therefore, the opportunity to develop suitable yeast strains for expressing human microsomal enzymes for the detection of the mutagenic activity of chemicals.

2.6 REFERENCES

Abt, K. (1981). Problems of repeated significance testing. *Controlled Clinical Trials*, **1**, 377–81.

Albertini, S., Friedrich, U., Gröschel-Stewart, U., Zimmermann, F. K. & Würgler, F. E. (1985). Phenobarbital induces aneuploidy in *Saccharomyces cerevisiae* and stimulates the assembly of porcine brain tubulin. *Mutation Research*, **144**, 67–71.

Albertini, S., Friederich, U. & Würgler, F. E. (1988). Induction of mitotic chromosome loss in the diploid yeast *Saccharomyces cerevisiae* D61.M by genotoxic carcinogens and tumor promoters. *Environ. Molec. Mutagenesis*, **11**, 497–508.

Ames, B. N., McCann, J. & Yamasaki, E. (1975). Methods for detecting carcinogens and mutagens with the *Salmonella*/mammalian microsome mutagenicity test. *Mutation Research*, **31**, 347–64.

Arlett, C. F., Smith, D. M., Green, M. H. L., McGregor, D. B., Clarke, G. M., Cole, J. & Asquith, J. C. (1989). Mammalian cell gene mutation assays based upon colony formation. In *Statistical Evaluation of Mutagenicity Test Data*, ed. D. J. Kirkland, Cambridge University Press, Cambridge, Chapter 3, pp. 66–101.

Baguley, B., Turner, P. M. & Ferguson, L. (1990). Protection by inhibitors of multidrug resistance against mitochondrial mutagenesis in *Saccharomyces cerevisiae*. *European Journal of Cancer*, **26**, 55–60.

Bartlett, M. S. (1947). The use of transformations. *Biometrics*, **3**, 39–52.

Black, S. M., Ellard, S., Meehan, R. R., Parry, J. M., Adesnik, M., Beggs, J. D. & Wolf, C. R. (1989). The expression of cytochrome P450IIB1 in *S. cerevisiae*. Results in an increased mutation frequency when exposed to cyclophosphamide. *Carcinogenesis*, **10**, 2139–43.

Blatiak, A. A., Gondal, J. A. & Wiseman, A. (1980). Mechanism of degradation of cyt. P450 in non-growing *S. cerevisiae*: Anaerobosis, chloramphenicol, dinitrophenol and cycloheximide as protective agents. *Biochemical Society Transactions*, **8**, 711–12.

Boguslawski, G. (1985). Effects of polymixin B nonapeptide on growth and permeability of the yeast *Saccharomyces cerevisiae*. *Molecular and General Genetics*, **199**, 401–5.

Box, G. E. P. & Cox, D. R. (1964). An analysis of transformations. *Journal of the Royal Statistical Society Series B*, **26**, 211–52.

Box, G. E. P. & Tiao, G. C. (1973). Inferences concerning the difference between two means. In *Bayesian Inference in Statistical Analysis*, Addison-Wesley, Reading, Massachusetts, Section 2.5, pp. 103–9.

Bradley, J. V. (1968). Normal scores tests. In *Distribution-free Statistical Tests*, Prentice-Hall Inc., Englewood Cliffs, NJ, Chapter 6, pp. 146–63 and Chapter 13, pp. 283–312.

Briza, P., Breitenbach, M., Ellinger, A. & Segall, J. (1990). Isolation of two developmentally regulated genes involved in spore wall maturation in *Saccharomyces cerevisiae*. *Genes and Development*, **4**, 1775–89.

Brusick, D. J. (1972). Induction of cycloheximide-resistant mutants in *Saccharomyces cerevisiae* with N-methyl-N'-nitro-N-nitrosoguanidine and ICR-170. *Journal of Bacteriology*, **109**, 1134–8.

Brusick, D. J. (1980). In *Principles of Genetic Toxicology*, Plenum Press, New York, Chapter 8, p. 201.

Brusick, D. J. & Andrews, H. (1974). Comparison of the genetic activity of dimethylnitrosamine, ethyl methanesulphonate, 2-acetylaminofluorene and ICR-170 in *Saccharomyces cerevisiae* straines D3, D4 and D5 using *in vitro* assays with and without metabolic activation. *Mutation Research*, **26**, 491–500.

Brusick, D. J. & Zeiger, E. (1972). A comparison of chemically induced reversion patterns of *Salmonella typhimurium* and *Saccharomyces cerevisiae* mutants, using *in vitro* plate tests. *Mutation Research*, **14**, 271–5.

Callen, D. F. (1981). Comparison of the genetic activity of AF-2 and nitro-furantoin in log and stationary phase cells of *Saccharomyces cerevisiae*. *Environmental Mutagenesis*, **3**, 641–58.

Callen, D. F. & Larson, R. A. (1978). Toxic and genetic effects of fuel oil photoproducts and three hydroperoxides in *Saccharomyces cerevisiae*. *Journal of Toxicology and Environmental Health*, **4**, 913–17.

Callen, D. F. & Philpott, R. M. (1977). Cytochrome P-450 and the activation of promutagens in *Saccharomyces cerevisiae*. *Mutation Research*, **45**, 309–24.

Callen, D. F., Wolf, C. R. & Philpott, R. M. (1980). Cytochrome P-450 mediated genetic activity and cytotoxicity of several halogenated aliphatic hydrocarbons in *Saccharomyces cerevisiae*. *Mutation Research*, **77**, 55–63.

Campbell, R. C. (1974*a*). Comparing several samples. In *Statistics for Biologists*, Cambridge University Press, Cambridge, Chapter 3, pp. 50–88.

Campbell, R. C. (1974*b*). Association. In *Statistics for Biologists*, Cambridge University Press, Cambridge, Chapter 4, pp. 89–114.

del Carratore, R., Bronzetti, G., Bauer, C., Corsi, C., Nieri, R., Paolini, M. & Gioagoni, P. (1983). Cytochrome P450 factors determining synthesis in strain D7 *Saccharomyces cerevisiae*. *Mutation Research*, **121**, 117–23.

Chattoo, B. B., Sherman, F., Azubalis, D. A., Fjellstedt, T. A., Mehnert, D. & Ogur, M. (1979). Selection of lys_2 mutants of the yeast *Saccharomyces cerevisiae* by the utilization of α-aminoadipate. *Genetics*, **93**, 51–65.

Ching, M. S., Lennard, M. S., Tucker, G. T., Woods, H. F., Kelly, D. E. & Kelly, S. L. (1991). The expression of human cytochrome PA501A1 in the yeast *Saccharomyces cerevisiae*. *Biochemical Pharmacology* (in press).

Davies, P. J. & Parry, J. M. (1976). The induction of mitotic gene conversion by chemical and physical mutagens as a function of culture age in the yeast, *Saccharomyces cerevisiae*. *Molecular and General Genetics*, **148**, 165–70.

de Serres, F. J. & Ashby, J. (eds.) (1981). In *Progress in Mutation Research: Evaluation of Short-term Tests for Carcinogens*, vol. 1, Elsevier, North Holland, New York.

Dixon, M. (1983). A yeast screening system for the detection of mutation, recombination and aneuploidy. US Dept. of Emergency Document LBL-16686.

Egilsson, N., Evans, I. H. & Wilkie, D. (1979). Toxic and mutagenic effects of carcinogens on the mitochondria of *Saccharomyces cerevisiae*. *Molecular and General Genetics*, **174**, 39–46.

Ephrussi, B. (1950). Induction par l'acriflavine d'une mutation specifique chez la levure. *Estratto dalle Publ. della Stazionne zool. di Napoli*. Suppl. al. Vol. XXII, 1–15.

Esposito, M. S., Maleas, D. T., Bjornstad, K. A. & Bruschi, C. V. (1982). Simultaneous detection of changes in chromosome number, gene conversion and intergenic recombination during meiosis of *Saccharomyces cerevisiae*: Spontaneous and ultraviolet light induced events. *Current Genetics*, **6**, 5–11.

Eugster, H. P., Friederich, V., Meyhack, B., Hinnen, A., Meyer, V. A. & Würgler, F. (1988). Modification of the D7 mutagenicity assay by heterologous expression of genes coding for xenobiotic metabolising enzymes. In *14th International Conference on Yeast Genetics and Molecular Biology.* John Wiley and Sons Ltd., p. 18.

Eugster, H. P., Sengstag, C., Meyer, V. A., Hinnen, A. & Würgler, F. E. (1990). Constitutive and inducible expression of human cytochrome P4501A1 in yeast *Saccharomyces cerevisiae*: An alternative source for *in vitro* studies. *Biochemical and Biophysical Research Communications,* **172,** 737–44.

Fabre, F. (1978). Induced intragenic recombination in yeast can occur during the G1 mitotic phase. *Nature,* **272,** 795–8.

Fahrig, R. (1976). The effect of dose and time on the induction of genetic alterations in *Saccharomyces cerevisiae* by aminoacridines in the presence and absence of visible light irradiation in comparison with the dose effect-curves of mutagens with other type of action. *Molecular and General Genetics,* **144,** 131–40.

Ferguson, L. R. (1984). Apparent changes in structure-activity relationship for antimitochondrial effects of 9-anilinoacridines according to *Saccharomyces cerevisiae* strain and methodology. *Mutation Research,* **136,** 223–31.

Ferguson, L. R. & Turner, P. M. (1988). Petite mutagenesis by anticancer drugs in *Saccharomyces cerevisiae. European Journal of Cancer Clinical Oncology,* **24,** 591–6.

Fogel, S. & Mortimer, R. K. (1969). Informational transfer in meiotic gene conversion. *Proceedings of the National Academy of Sciences, USA,* **62,** 96–103.

Garde, J. (1986). Studies upon the induction of chromosome aneuploidy in eukaryotic cells. PhD Thesis, University of Wales.

Gilberg, B. O. & Aman, J. (1971). Petite mutants induced in yeast by optical brighteners. *Mutation Research,* **13,** 149–54.

Grenson, M., Mousset, M., Wiame, J. M. & Bechet, J. (1966). Multiplicity of the amino-acid permeases in *Saccharomyces cerevisiae. Biochimica et Biophysica Acta,* **127,** 325–38.

Hartwell, L. H. (1974). *Saccharomyces cerevisiae* cell cycle. *Bacterial Reviews,* **38,** 164–98.

Hrelia, P., Murelli, L., Paolini, M., Sapigni, E. & Cantelli-Forti, G. (1987). Inducibility of NADPH cytochrome c(P450) reductase in yeast: role in the bioactivation of nitroimidazo (2,1-b)triazoles. *Mutagenesis,* **2,** 425–9.

Imai, Y. (1988). Characterization of rabbit liver cytochrome P-450 (laurate w-1 hydroxylase) synthesized in transformed yeast cells. *Journal of Biochemistry,* **103,** 143–8.

Iwamoto, Y., Yanagihara, Y., Yielding, L. W. & Yielding, K. L. (1986). Petite induction in yeast, *Saccharomyces cerevisiae*, by phenanthridinium compounds: Promotive effects of propidium iodide on mutagenesis by ethidium bromide or 8-deaminoethidium chloride. *Chemical and Pharmaceutical Bulletin,* **34,** 1735–9.

Jagannath, D. R., Brusick, D. J., Everett, D. & Lacivita, C. L. (1985). Genetic activity of mycotoxin, sterigmatocystin in yeast assays. *Environmental Mutagenesis,* **7** (3), 59.

Jagannath, D. R., Vultaggio, D. M. and Brusick, D. J. (1981). Genetic activity of 42 coded compounds in the mitotic gene conversion assay using *Saccharomyces cerevisiae* strain D4. In *Progress in Mutation Research,* vol. 1, eds. F. J. de Serres and J. Ashby. Elsevier, North Holland, New York, Chapter 41, pp. 456–67.

Kalb, V. F., Loper, J. C., Dey, C. R., Woods, C. W. & Sutter, T. R. (1986). Isolation of a cytochrome P-450 structural gene from *Saccharomyces cerevisiae. Gene*, **45**, 237–45.

Kastenbaum, M. A. & Bowman, K. O. (1970). Tables for determining the statistical significance of mutation frequencies. *Mutation Research*, **9**, 527–49.

Kelly, D. E. & Parry, J. M. (1983). Metabolic activation by cytochrome P450/P448 in the yeast *Saccharomyces cerevisiae. Mutation Research*, **108**, 147–58.

Kilbey, B. J. & Zetterberg, G. (1973). A re-examination of the genetic effects of optical brighteners in yeast. *Mutation Research*, **21**, 73–82.

Koch, R., Schlegelmilch, R. & Wolf, H. U. (1988). Genetic effects of chlorinated ethylenes in the yeast *Saccharomyces cerevisiae. Mutation Research*, **206**, 209–16.

Kunz, B. A., Barclay, B. J. & Haynes, R. H. (1980). A simple, rapid plate assay for mitotic recombination. *Mutation Research*, **73**, 215–50.

Kunz, B. A. & Haynes, R. H. (1982). DNA repair and the genetic effects of thymidylate stress in yeast. *Mutation Research*, **93**, 353–75.

Lawrence, C. W. (1982). Mutagenesis in *Saccharomyces cerevisiae. Advances in Genetics*, **21**, 173–254.

Leadbeater, L. & Davis, D. R. (1964). Stability of enzymes of liver microsomal preparations. *Biochemical Pharmacology*, **13**, 1609–17.

Lemontt, J. F. (1977). Mutagenesis of yeast by hydrazine: dependence upon post-treatment cell division. *Mutation Research*, **43**, 165–78.

Lindenmayer, A. & Smith, L. (1964). Cytochromes and other pigments of baker's yeast grown aerobically and anaerobically. *Biochimica et Biophysica Acta*, **93**, 445–61.

Loprieno, N. (1981). Screening of coded carcinogenic and noncarcinogenic chemicals by a forward mutation system with the yeast *Schizosaccharomyces pombe*. In *Progress in Mutation Research*, vol. 1, eds. F. J. de Serres and J. Ashby, Elsevier, North Holland, New York, Chapter 39, pp. 424–33.

Lovell, D. P. (1989). Statistics and genetic toxicology – setting the scene. In *Statistical Evaluation of Mutagenicity Test Data*, ed. D. J. Kirkland, Cambridge University Press, Cambridge, Chapter 1, pp. 1–25.

Mahon, G. A. T., Middleton, B., Robinson, W. D., Green, M. H. L., Mitchell, I. deG. & Tweats, D. J. (1989). Analysis of data from microbial colony assays. In *Statistical Evaluation of Mutagenicity Test Data*, ed. D. J. Kirkland, Cambridge University Press, Cambridge, Chapter 2, pp. 26–65.

Mayer, V. W. & Goin, C. J. (1987). Aneuploidy induced by nocodazole or ethyl acetate is suppressed by dimethyl sulfoxide. *Mutation Research*, **187**, 31–5.

Mayer, V. W. & Goin, C. J. (1989). Observations on chromosome loss detection by multiple recessive marker expression in strain D61.M of *Saccharomyces cerevisiae. Mutation Research*, **224**, 471–8.

Mayer, V. W., Goin, C. J. & Zimmermann, F. K. (1986). Aneuploidy and other genetic effects induced by hydroxyurea in *Saccharomyces cerevisiae. Mutation Research*, **160**, 19–26.

Mayer, V. W., Hybner, C. J. & Brusick, D. J. (1976). Genetic effects induced by *Saccharomyces cerevisiae* by cyclophosphamide *in vitro* without liver enzyme preparations. *Mutation Research*, **37**, 201–12.

Mehta, R. D. & von Borstel, R. C. (1981). Mutagenic activity of 42 encoded compounds in the haploid reversion strain XV185-14C. In *Progress in*

Mutation Research, vol. 1, eds. F. J. de Serres and J. Ashby. Elsevier, North Holland, New York, Chapter 38, pp. 414–23.

Mehta, R. D. & von Borstel, R. C. (1985). Tests for genetic activity in the yeast *Saccharomyces cerevisiae* using strains D7-144, XV185-14C and RM52. In *Progress in Mutation Research*, vol. 5, eds. F. J. de Serres and J. Ashby. Elsevier, North Holland, New York, Chapter 23, pp. 271–84.

Mitchell, I. de G. (1987). The interaction of statistical significance, biology of dose–response and test design in the assessment of genotoxicity data. *Mutagenesis*, **2**, 141–75.

Mitchell, I. de G., Dixon, P. A., Gilbert, P. J. & White, D. J. (1980). Mutagenicity of antibiotics in microbial assays: problems of evaluation. *Mutation Research*, **79**, 91–105.

Mitchell, I. de G. & Gilbert, P. J. (1984). The effect of pretreatment of *Escherichia coli* CM891 with ethylenediaminetetraacetate on sensitivity to a variety of standard mutagens. *Mutation Research*, **140**, 13–19.

Mitchell, I. de G. & Gilbert, P. J. (1985). Gene mutation in yeast induced by DAB, CDA, BZD and DAT. In *Comparative Genetic Toxicology*, eds. J. M. Parry and C. F. Arlett, MacMillan Press, Basingstoke, Chapter 29, pp. 241–52.

Mitchell, I. de G. & Gilbert, P. J. (1991). Comparison of forward mutation at the cycloheximide, canavanine and adipic acid resistance loci in response to treatment of wild type *Saccharomyces cerevisiae* strain S7a with eight polycyclic aromatic compounds. *Mutagenesis*, **6**, 229–36.

Mitchell, I. de G., Rees, R. W., Gilbert, P. J. & Carlton, J. B. (1990). The use of historical data for identifying biologically unimportant but statistically significant results in genotoxicity assays. *Mutagenesis*, **5**, 159–64.

Moore, C. W. (1978). Bleomycin-induced mutation and recombination in *Saccharomyces cerevisiae*. *Mutation Research*, **58**, 41–9.

Morita, T., Iwamoto, Y., Shimizu, T., Masuzawa, T. & Yanagihara, Y. (1989). Mutagenicity tests with a permeable mutant of yeast on carcinogens showing false-negative in Salmonella assay. *Chemical and Pharmacological Bulletin*, **37**, 407–9.

Murphy, S. A., Caspary, W. J. & Margolin, B. H. (1988). A statistical analysis for the mouse lymphoma cell forward mutation assay. *Mutation Research*, **203**, 145–54.

Murthy, M. S. S. (1979). Induction of gene conversion in diploid yeast by chemicals: correlation with mutagenic action and its relevance in geno-toxicity screening. *Mutation Research*, **64**, 1–17.

Nebert, D., Adesnik, M., Coon, M. J., Estabrook, R. W., Gonzalez, F. J., Guengerich, F. P., Gunsalus, I. C., Johnson, E. F., Kemper, B., Levin, W., Phillips, I. R., Sato, R. & Waterman, M. R. (1987). The P450 gene super-family: Recommended nomenclature. *DNA*, **6**, 1–11.

Nebert, D., Nelson, D. R., Coon, M. J., Estabrook, R. W., Feyereisen, R., Fujii-Kuriyama, Y., Gonzalez, F. J., Guengerich, F. P., Gunsalus, I. C., Johnson, E. F., Loper, J. C., Sato, R., Waterman, M. R. & Waxman, D. J. (1991). The P450 superfamily: Update on new sequences, gene mapping, and recommended nomenclature. *DNA and Cell Biology*, **10**, 1–14.

Niggli, B., Friederich, U., Hann, D. & Würgler, F. E. (1986). Endogenous promutagen activation in the yeast *Saccharomyces cerevisiae*: factors influencing aflatoxin B$_1$ mutagenicity. *Mutation Research*, **175**, 223–9.

Niggli, B., Friederich, U. & Würgler, F. E. (1988). Endogenous activation of Aflatoxin B1 in the yeast *Saccharomyces cerevisiae* D7: factors influencing mutagenicity and P450 content. *Mutation Research*, **203**, 209–10.

Oeda, K., Sakaki, T. & Ohkawa, H. (1985). Expression of rat liver cytochrome P-450MC cDNA in *Saccharomyces cerevisiae*. *DNA*, **4**, 203–10.

Ogur, M., John, R. S. & Nagai, S. (1957). Tetrazolium overlay technique for population studies of respiration deficiency in yeast. *Science*, **125**, 928–9.

Paolini, M., Sapigni, E., Hrelia, P., Grilli, S., Lattanzi, G., Scotti, M. & Cantelli Forti, G. (1990). Strategies for optimization of short-term genotoxicity tests: the synergistic effect of NADPH and NADH on P450 function in processing pre-mutagens. *Mutagenesis*, **5**, 51–4.

Parry, E. M. & Parry J. M. (1984). The assay of genotoxicity of chemicals using the budding yeast *Saccharomyces cerevisiae*. In *Mutagenicity testing: A practical Approach*, eds. S. Venitt and J. M. Parry. IRL Press, Oxford, Chapter 5, pp. 119–47.

Parry, J. M. (1977). The use of yeast cultures for the detection of environmental mutagens using a fluctuation test. *Mutation Research*, **46**, 165–76.

Parry, J. M. (1982). The effects of BC, 4CMB and 4HMB upon the induction of mitotic gene conversion in yeast. *Mutation Research*, **100**, 145–51.

Parry, J. M., Davies, P. J. & Evans, W. E. (1976). The effects of 'cell age' upon the lethal effects of physical and chemical mutagens in the yeast, *Saccharomyces cerevisiae*. *Molecular and General Genetics*, **146**, 27–35.

Parry, J. M. & Eckardt, F. (1985*a*). The detection of mitotic gene conversion, point mutation and mitotic segregation using the yeast *Saccharomyces cerevisiae* strain D7. In *Progress in Mutation Research*, vol. 5, eds. J. Ashby and F. J. de Serres. Elsevier Sciences Publishers, Amsterdam, Chapter 22, pp. 261–9.

Parry, J. M. & Eckardt, F. (1985*b*). The induction of mitotic aneuploidy, point mutation and mitotic crossing-over in the yeast *Saccharomyces cerevisiae* strains D61-M and D6. In *Progress in Mutation Research*, vol. 5, eds. J. Ashby and F. J. de Serres. Elsevier Science Publishers, Amsterdam, Chapter 24, pp. 285–95.

Parry, J. M., Parry, E. M., Warr, T., Lynch, A. & James S. (1990). The detection of aneugens using yeast and cultured mammalian cells. In *Mutation and the Environment, Part B*, eds. M. Mendelsohn and R. A. Albertini, Wiley Liss Inc., pp. 247–66.

Parry, J. M. & Sharp D. C. (1981). Induction of mitotic aneuploidy in the yeast strain D6 by 42 coded compounds. In *Progress in Mutation Research*, vol. 1, eds. F. J. de Serres and J. Ashby. Elsevier, North Holland, Chapter 42, pp. 468–80.

Parry, J. M., Sharp, D. & Parry, E. M. (1979). Detection of mitotic and meiotic aneuploidy in the yeast *Saccharomyces cerevisiae*. *Environmental Health Perspectives*, **31**, 97–111.

Parry, J. M. & Zimmermann, F. K. (1976). The detection of monosome colonies produced by mitotic chromosome non-disjunction in the yeast *Saccharomyces cerevisiae*. *Mutation Research*, **36**, 49–66.

Patel, R. & Wilkie, D. (1982). Mitochondrial toxicity in Saccharomyces as a measure of carcinogenicity. *Mutation Research*, **100**, 179–83.

Piegorsch, W. W., Zimmermann, F. K., Fogel, S., Whittaker, S. G. & Resnick, A. (1989). Quantitative approaches for assessing chromosome loss in *Saccharomyces cerevisiae*: general methods for analyzing downturns in dose response. *Mutation Research*, **224**, 11–29.

Rees, R. W., Brice, A. J., Carlton, J. B., Gilbert, P. J. & Mitchell, I. de G. (1989). Optimization of metabolic activation for four mutagens in a bacterial, fungal and two mammalian cell mutagenesis assays. *Mutagenesis*, **4**, 335–42.

Resnick, M. A., Mayer, V. M. & Zimmermann, F. K. (1986). The detection of chemically induced aneuploidy in *Saccharomyces cerevisiae*: an assessment of mitotic and meiotic systems. *Mutation Research*, **167**, 47–60.

Resnick, M. A., Skaanild, M. & Nilsson-Tillgren, T. (1989). Lack of DNA homology in a pair of divergent chromosomes greatly sensitizes them to loss by DNA damage. *Proceedings of the National Academy of Sciences, USA*, **86**, 2276–80.

Robinson, W. D., Green, M. H. L., Cole, J., Garner, R. C., Healy, M. J. R. & Gatehouse, D. (1989). Statistical evaluation of bacterial/mammalian fluctuation test. In *Statistical Evaluation of Mutagenicity Test Data*, ed. D. J. Kirkland, Cambridge University Press, Cambridge, Chapter 4, pp. 102–40.

Rockmill, B. & Fogel, S. (1988). DIS1: a yeast gene required for proper meiotic chromosome disjunction. *Genetics*, **119**, 261–72.

Roman, H. (1956). A system selective for mutations affecting the synthesis of adenine in yeast. *Comptes Rendus des Travaux du Laboratoire Carlesberg Serie Physiologie*, **26**, 299–314.

Sankaranarayanan, N. & Murthy, M. S. S. (1979). Testing of some permitted food colors for the induction of gene conversion in diploid yeast *Saccharomyces cerevisiae. Mutation Research*, **67**, 309–14.

Schiestl, R. H. (1989). Nonmutagenic carcinogens induce intrachromosomal recombination in yeast. *Nature*, **337**, 285–8.

Schiestl, R. H., Gretz, R. D., Mehta, R. D. & Hastings, P. J. (1989). Carcinogens induce intrachromosomal recombination in yeast. *Carcinogenesis*, **10**, 1445–55.

Schiestl, R. H., Igarashi, S. & Hastings, P. J. (1988). Analysis of the mechanism for reversion of a disrupted gene. *Genetics*, **119**, 237–47.

Shahin, M. M. (1975). Genetic activity of niridazole in yeast. *Mutation Research*, **30**, 191–8.

Shahin, M. M. & von Borstel, R. C. (1978). Comparisons of mutation induction in reversion systems of *Saccharomyces cerevisiae* and *Salmonella typhimurium. Mutation Research*, **53**, 1–10.

Sharp, D. C. & Parry, J. M. (1981). Induction of mitotic gene conversion by 41 coded compounds using the yeast cultures JD1. In *Progress in Mutation Research*, vol. 1, eds. F. J. de Serres and J. Ashby. Elsevier, North Holland, New York, Chapter 44, pp. 491–501.

Shay, J. W. & Werbin, H. (1987). Are mitochondrial DNA mutations involved in the carcinogenic process? *Mutation Research*, **186**, 149–60.

Siebert, D., Bayer, U. & Marquardt, H. (1979). The application of mitotic gene conversion in *Saccharomyces cerevisiae* in a pattern of four assays *in vitro* and *in vivo*, for mutagenicity testing. *Mutation Research*, **67**, 145–56.

Snedecor, G. W. & Cochran, W. G. (1967). Test for a linear trend in proportions. In *Statistical Methods*, 6th edn. Iowa State University Press, Section 9.11, pp. 246–7.

Sora, S. (1985). Effects of some DNA-ligands and of some mutagenic compounds on the induction of meiotic disomic or diploid yeast products. *Environmental Mutagenesis*, **7**, 121–8.

Sora, S. & Magni, G. E. (1988). Induction of meiotic chromosomal malsegregation in yeast. *Mutation Research*, **201**, 375–84.

Sora, S., Lucchini, G. & Magni, G. E. (1982). Meiotic diploid progeny and meiotic non-disjunction in *Saccharomyces cerevisiae*. *Genetics*, **101**, 17–33.

Sora, S., Crippa, M. & Lucchini, G. (1983). Disomic and diploid meiotic products in *Saccharomyces cerevisiae*. Effect of vincristine, vinblastine, adriamycin, bleomycin, mitomycin C, and cyclophosphamide. *Mutation Research*, **197**, 249–64.

Stansfield, I., Cliffe, K. & Kelly, S. L. (1991). Chemostat studies of microsomal enzyme induction in *Saccharomyces cerevisiae*. *Yeast*, **7**, 147–56.

Thacker, J. (1974). An assessment of ultrasonic radiation hazard using yeast genetic systems. *British Journal Radiobiology*, **47**, 130–8.

Urban, P., Cullin, C. & Pompon, D. (1990). Maximising the expression of mammalian cytochrome P450 monooxygenase activities in yeast cells. *Biochimie*, **72**, 463–72.

Von Borstel, R. C. & Quah, S. K. (1973). Induction of mutations in *Saccharomyces* with hycanthone. *Mutation Research*, **21**, 52.

Whittaker, S. G., Rockmill, B. M., Blechl, A. E., Malony, D. H., Resnick, M. A. & Fogel, S. (1988). The detection of mitotic and meiotic aneuploidy in yeast using a gene dosage selection system. *Molecular and General Genetics*, **215**, 10–18.

Whittaker, S. G., Zimmermann, F. K., Dicus, B., Piegorsch, W. W., Fogel, S. & Resnick, M. A. (1989). Detection of induced mitotic chromosome loss in *Saccharomyces cerevisiae* – an interlaboratory study. *Mutation Research*, **224**, 31–78.

Whittaker, S. G., Zimmermann, F. K., Dicus, B., Piegorsch, W. W., Resnick, M. A. & Fogel, S. (1990*a*). Detection of induced mitotic chromosome loss in *Saccharomyces cerevisiae* – an interlaboratory assessment of 12 chemicals. *Mutation Research*, **241**, 225–42.

Whittaker, S. G., Moser, S. F., Maloney, D. H., Piegorsch, W. W., Resnick, M. A. & Fogel, S. (1990*b*). The detection of mitotic and meiotic chromosome gain in the yeast *Saccharomyces cerevisiae*: effects of methyl benzimidazol-2-yl-carbamate, methyl methanesulfonate, ethyl methanesulfonate, dimethyl sulfoxide, propionitrile and cyclophosphamide monohydrate. *Mutation Research*, **242**, 231–58.

Wilcox, P. (1984). Studies in Genetic Toxicology. PhD Thesis, University of Wales.

Wilkie, D., Evans, I. H., Egilsson, V., Diala, E. S. & Collier, D. (1983). Mitochondria, cell surface and carcinogenesis. *International Reviews in Cytology*, Supplement 15, 157–89.

Wiseman, A., Lim, T.-K. & McCloud, C. (1975*a*). Relationship of cytochrome P450 to growth phase of brewers yeast in 1% or 20% glucose medium. *Biochemical Society Transactions*, **3**, 276–8.

Wiseman, A., Gondal, J. A. & Sims, P. (1975*b*). 4'-hydroxylation of biphenyl by yeast containing cyt.P450: radiation and thermal stability, comparisons with liver enzyme. *Biochemical Society Transactions*, **3**, 278–81.

Wiseman, A., Jay, F. & Gondal, J. A. (1975*c*). Metabolism of xenobiotics by intact brewers yeast containing cyt.P450. *Journal of Science of Food and Agriculture*, **26**, 539–40.

Yabusaki, Y., Murakami, H. & Ohkawa, H. (1988). Primary structure of *Saccharomyces cerevisiae* NADPH-cytochrome P450 reductase deducted from nucleotide sequence of its cloned gene. *Journal of Biochemistry*, **103**, 1004–10.

Yasumori, T., Murayama, N., Yamazoe, Y., Aloe, A., Nogi, Y., Fukasawa, T. & Kato, R. (1989). Expression of a human P450IIC gene in yeast cells using galatose-inducible expression system. *Molecular Pharmacology*, **35**, 443–9.

Yoshida, Y. & Aoyama, Y. (1984). Yeast cytochrome P450 catalyzing lanosterol 14 α-demethylation. I. Purification and spectral properties. *Journal of Biological Chemistry*, **259**, 1655–60.

Zetterberg, G. (1979). Mechanism of the lethal and mutagenic effects of phenoxyacetic acids in *Saccharomyces cerevisiae*. *Mutation Research*, **60**, 291–300.

Zetterberg, G. & Bostrom, G. (1981). Mitotic gene conversion induced in yeast by isoniazid. Influence of a transition metal and of the physiological conditions of the cells. *Mutation Research*, **91**, 215–19.

Zimmermann, F. K. (1969). Genetic effects of polynuclear hydrocarbons: Induction of mitotic gene conversion. *Zeitschrift Krebsforsch*, **72**, 65–71.

Zimmermann, F. K. (1971). Induction of mitotic gene conversion by mutagens. *Mutation Research*, **11**, 327–37.

Zimmermann, F. K. (1973*a*). Detection of genetically active chemicals using various yeast systems. In *Chemical Mutagens. Principles and Methods for Their Detection*, vol. 3, ed. Hollaender, Plenum Press, New York, pp. 209–39.

Zimmermann, F. K. (1973*b*). A yeast strain for visual screening for the two reciprocal products of mitotic crossing-over. *Mutation Research*, **21**, 263–9.

Zimmermann, F. K. (1975). Procedures used in the induction of mitotic recombination and mutation in the yeast *Saccharomyces cerevisiae*. *Mutation Research*, **31**, 71–86.

Zimmermann, F. K., Kern, R. & Rasenberger, H. (1975). A yeast strain for simultaneous detection of induced mitotic crossing-over, mitotic gene conversion and reverse mutation. *Mutation Research*, **28**, 381–8.

Zimmermann, F. K. & Scheel, I. (1981). Induction of mitotic gene conversion in strain D7 of *Saccharomyces cerevisiae* by 42 coded chemicals. In *Progress in Mutation Research*, vol. 1, eds. F. J. de Serres and J. Ashby. Elsevier, North Holland, New York, Chapter 43, pp. 481–90.

Zimmermann, F. K., Mayer, V. W. & Parry, J. M. (1982). Genetic toxicology studies using *Saccharomyces cerevisiae*. *Journal of Applied Toxicology*, **2**, 1–10.

Zimmermann, F. K., Mayer, V. W. & Scheel, I. (1984*a*). Induction of aneuploidy by oncodazole (nocodazole), an anti-tubulin agent, and acetone. *Mutation Research*, **141**, 15–18.

Zimmermann, F. K., von Borstel, R. C., Parry, J. M., Stieberg, D., Zetterberg, G., von Halle, E. S., Barale, R. & Loprieno, N. (1984*b*). Testing of chemicals for genetic activity with *Saccharomyces cerevisiae*: report of the US Environmental Protection Agency Gene-Tox Program. *Mutation Research*, **133**, 199–244.

Zimmermann, F. K. & Scheel, I. (1984). Genetic effects of 5-azacytidine in *Saccharomyces cerevisiae*. *Mutation Research*, **139**, 21–4.

Zimmermann, F. K., Gröschel-Stewart, U., Scheel, I. & Resnick, M. A. (1985*a*). Genetic change may be caused by interference with protein–protein interactions. *Mutation Research*, **150**, 203–10.

Zimmermann, F. K., Mayer, V. M., Scheel, I. & Resnick, M. A. (1985*b*). Acetone, methyl ethyl ketone, ethyl acetate, acetonitrile and other polar aprotic solvents are strong inducers of aneuploidy in *Saccharomyces cerevisiae*. *Mutation Research*, **149**, 339–51.

Zimmermann, F. K., Henning, H. J., Scheel, I. & Oehler, M. (1986). Genetic and anti-tubulin effects induced by pyridine derivatives. *Mutation Research*, **163**, 23–31.

3

In vivo rat liver UDS assay

J. C. Kennelly   R. Waters   J. Ashby
P. A. Lefevre   B. Burlinson   D. J. Benford
S. W. Dean   I. de G. Mitchell

3.1   INTRODUCTION

3.1.1   Objective

In the first edition *UKEMS Part II Guidelines* Waters *et al.* (1984) described the theory and practice of assays for unscheduled DNA synthesis (UDS). Since then, there has been extensive development of the rat *in vivo* liver UDS assay and it was considered timely to update the UDS section of the UKEMS guidelines, concentrating on the *in vivo* rat liver UDS assay. This also is an opportunity to include procedures and modifications that have arisen since the publication of the ASTM guideline for the *in vivo* rat liver UDS assay (Butterworth *et al.*, 1987).

3.1.2   Application of *in vivo* genotoxicity tests

When testing for genotoxicity, the use of *in vitro* methods presents problems that may be intractable given the nature of the systems employed. In an *in vitro* system, reactions yielding a DNA reactive species may only occur under conditions that do not apply to the whole animal *in vivo*. Furthermore, in the whole animal, the dynamics of absorption, distribution, metabolism including detoxification and excretion may prevent activated metabolites achieving target tissue concentrations likely to cause any significant effects. Consideration of *in vitro* genotoxicity data alone will therefore give rise to a number of false assignments with respect to *in vivo* genotoxic activity. To improve the predictive value of testing programmes the strategic use of *in vivo* tests, including the rat liver UDS assay, enables a realistic assessment of mutagenic hazard (Ashby, 1983).

The guidelines of the UK Department of Health's Committee on Mutagenicity of Chemicals in Food Consumer Products and the Environment (Department of Health, 1989) recognise the important role of *in vivo* genotoxicity testing in assessment of potential mutagenic risk. The principal role of such studies is in assessing whether compounds identified as having mutagenic potential *in vitro* can express this activity in the whole animal. In the first instance, a bone marrow assay for clastogenic damage is recommended, such as the well-established mouse micronucleus assay. UKEMS have recently published revised procedures for these assays (Richold *et al.*, 1990). A negative result in a bone marrow assay on its own, however, is insufficient to provide reassurance that activity cannot be expressed *in vivo* and data from at least one other tissue are necessary. It is therefore appropriate to apply a complementary *in vivo* assay system using a different organ. The liver, as the major organ of xenobiotic metabolism is an appropriate target in an assay for induced *in vivo* genetic effects and complements established assays using peripheral tissues such as the bone marrow. The *in vivo* rat liver UDS assay, primarily by virtue of examining a different target organ, may respond to many of the genotoxins undetected by the micronucleus assay (Ashby, 1986). In most cases where the bone marrow assay is in the mouse, the use of the rat liver UDS assay also complements by providing an assay in a second species. In recent years, the *in vivo* rat liver UDS assay has gained a wider acceptance for this role in assessment of genotoxic hazard (Department of Health, 1989).

The rat liver UDS assay is therefore used in a second, *in vivo*, tier of genotoxicity testing. In most cases, compounds will have already been tested *in vitro* to define their genotoxic potential. To evaluate whether this potential is expressed *in vivo*, it is usual to test in a mouse micronucleus assay. If the micronucleus test proves negative, the compound may be tested in the rat liver UDS assay.

3.1.3 UDS assays

UDS assays measure the resultant excision repair of DNA following a permanent change, such as the covalent binding of an activated mutagen or a reactive chemical species generated intracellularly, or the products of chemical events following ionising radiation damage (Rassmusson & Painter, 1964). Characteristically, the cell undergoing DNA repair processes will synthesise DNA at stages of the cell cycle other than S phase, where normal replicative or 'scheduled' DNA synthesis takes place, hence the term 'unscheduled' DNA synthesis for these repair phenomena (Djordjevic & Tolmach, 1967). Details of assays based on UDS have been described by Waters *et al.* (1984).

The magnitude of the UDS response is dependent on the number of DNA bases excised and replaced following damage. This may show poor correlation with the number of lesions; for example, X-irradiation produces a low level of UDS/lesion, i.e. 'short patch repair', where 1–3 bases are replaced, while UV produces high levels of UDS, 'long patch repair' with 20–40 bases replaced/ lesion (Regan & Setlow, 1974; Hanawalt *et al.*, 1979). Furthermore, mutagenic events may result because of non-repair, misrepair or misreplication of DNA lesions. The extent of the UDS response gives no indication of the fidelity of the repair process. In theory, it is possible that a mutagen may react with DNA, but undergo repair solely by post-replication and recombination-type repair mechanisms and so be undetected (Fox, 1988). The lack of specific information on comparative mutagenic/carcinogenic potential provided by UDS tests is compensated for by the potential sensitivity of an endpoint where the whole genome is the possible target for chemical reaction and repair.

UDS assays have been used for a number of years in screening programmes for mutagenic activity usually employing the measurement of induction of UDS following chemical treatment *in vitro* of transformed cell lines or primary cultures of hepatocytes. The value of UDS as an endpoint is that it is a consequence of direct or indirect chemical reaction with DNA so should not respond to compounds that affect DNA by other mechanisms, for example non-covalently bound intercalating agents (Waters *et al.*, 1984). Recently, there has been increasing use of UDS as an indicator of induced genetic effects in various tissues of animals treated with a compound *in vivo* (for review see Furihata & Matsushima, 1987). Of these, the most widely used *in vivo* UDS technique is the rat liver UDS assay.

3.1.4   *In vivo* rat liver UDS

The potential value of using an *in vivo* treatment coupled with an *in vitro* determination of UDS was described by Stich and Kieser (1974). In their technique, several organs of mice, including liver, were examined for UDS following injection of animals with dimethyl nitrosamine, 4-nitro-quinoline-1-oxide (NQO) or the non-carcinogenic metabolite of NQO, 4-aminoquinoline-1-oxide. Here the *in vivo* UDS response in various tissues correlated with the organ-specific carcinogenic action of the test compounds.

Measurement of UDS in hepatocyte cultures was developed as a screening assay for genotoxins *in vitro* by Williams (Williams, 1976, 1977, 1978; Williams & Laspia, 1979; Williams, Laspia & Dunkel, 1982). This assay was modified by Mirsalis and Butterworth (1980) for measurement of *in vivo* genotoxic activity. Animals receive the test agent *in vivo*, then primary hepatocyte cultures from these animals are examined for UDS induction using established *in vitro* methods.

The *in vitro* hepatocyte UDS test and *in vivo* rat liver UDS assay have different specificities. Some compounds, such as benzo(a)pyrene, are active when directly applied to hepatocyte cultures *in vitro* (Probst *et al.*, 1981) but no effect is detectable in the liver after dosage of the whole animal *in vivo* (Mirsalis, Tyson & Butterworth, 1982) at least by the standard single-dose protocol (Puri & Müller, 1989). In such cases, the net effect of whole body distribution and metabolism prevents any detectable liver DNA damage. Conversely, some mutagens may require specific *in vivo* biotransformation, e.g.: conjugation or metabolism by intestinal microflora for activity, so pass undetected in the *in vitro* hepatocyte assay. For example, the hepatocarcinogen 2,6 dinitrotoluene is negative in the *in vitro* hepatocyte UDS assay, but positive when tested for induction of UDS *in vivo* (Bermudez, Tillery & Butterworth, 1979; Mirsalis & Butterworth, 1982). In this particular instance, nitroreduction by gut microflora is an essential step in the metabolic activation of the compound to a DNA-reactive species.

3.1.5   Recommended methods for quantifying UDS
Currently there are two main methods of quantifying UDS. Both rely on the uptake of radiolabelled nucleotides, usually [^{3}H]thymidine, during DNA repair. The radiolabelling of DNA can be quantified either by extraction and determination of specific radioactivity by spectrophotometry and scintillation counting, or by microautoradiographs of cell preparations.

The use of scintillation counting presents particular problems as the specific radioactivity of DNA in S phase cells will be many times that of DNA in cells undergoing UDS. The presence of S phase cells could therefore invalidate the whole procedure. In order to apply the scintillation counting method, as is commonly used with cell lines such as HeLa, replicative DNA synthesis is suppressed by, e.g. growing to confluency, deprivation of serum and essential amino acids and the presence of hydroxyurea (Martin, McDermid & Garner, 1978). The scintillation counting method is rapid and considerably less labour intensive than a comparable method using autoradiography. There remains the concern that a test chemical which, for example, inhibited the hydroxyurea block could generate an apparent increase in UDS merely by allowing S phase to proceed in a greater fraction of the treated cell population compared with the negative control. The full range of S phase suppression techniques is not available for a primary cell culture system such as hepatocytes, and the action of hydroxyurea alone does not completely abolish S phase activity in whole liver (Reitz *et al.*, 1980), or in hepatocyte cultures (Glauert *et al.*, 1985). Furthermore, it is also likely that the proportion of cells in S phase will vary significantly between cultures derived from different animals. For these reasons, the use of scintillation counting is not recommended for determination of *in vivo* liver UDS, rather autoradiographic methods (Cleaver & Thomas, 1981) should be employed instead.

In microautoradiographic techniques, cell preparations previously exposed to radiolabelled nucleotide are covered with a layer of photographic emulsion sensitive to the emission of radioactive particles. Where emission of a particle has occurred, chemical reaction deposits metallic silver which is visualised as a discrete dark particle (grain) within the emulsion layer after development. The number of grains over areas of the cell may be scored by microscope. The number of grains over the nucleus compared with those over the cytoplasm provide a quantitative measurement of radiolabelling, hence of DNA synthesis. Cells undergoing normal S phase DNA synthesis prior to cell division are clearly recognised, as their nuclei appear black due to the presence of innumerable silver grains. Cells exhibiting UDS show more moderate increases in nuclear radiolabelling compared with controls.

Chemically induced increases in S phase activity have the potential to cause problems even in autoradiographic assays. In such circumstances, the proportion of cells which had taken up a small amount of radiolabel at the beginning of S phase could be increased and mistaken for cells in UDS. In practice, however, this confusion does not occur. Ashby *et al.* (1986) examined autoradiograms of hepatocytes sampled 36 hours after treatment with 1000 mg/kg of the mitogen 4-acetylaminofluorine (4-AAF). These showed a marked increase in S phase cells (10% incidence compared with 0.14% in solvent controls), however measured levels of UDS in apparent non-S phase cells were identical in negative control and treated groups. Similarly, induction of S phase by N-nitrosodibenzylamine gave no apparent increase in UDS (Schmetzer *et al.*, 1990).

Typical rat hepatocyte autoradiographs are shown in Fig. 3.1.

3.2   TEST MATERIALS
3.2.1   Test animals

The development of the assay was with male rats and this is the test animal with the largest database. Several strains of rats have been used; the Fischer 344, Wistar, Alderley Park and PVG animals. No significant qualitative strain differences in response to reference carcinogens have been reported. Some of the observed quantitative differences in solvent control values between laboratories have been associated with the use of different strains (Margolin & Risko, 1988). The use of female rats (Mirsalis & Butterworth, 1982) or other rodent species is rare and it is advised that the routine use of other than male rats should only be applied when a laboratory has accumulated a suitable database. Animals should be housed appropriately and allowed free access to food and water during the period of experiment.

3.2.2   Test agent

The following data should be available for the test agent where possible: i) Purity as percentage active ingredient and identity of major impurities, ii) solubility in solvents suitable for animal dosage, iii) stability in the chosen dosing vehicle should be considered, iv) chemical structure, this will enable comparison with structurally related compounds and the choice of chemical class controls, if appropriate, v) safety information (this will identify any particular handling procedures or other toxicological hazard, although all test agents are handled assuming they are potentially carcinogenic).

Where possible, test compounds should be dissolved in water or isotonic saline. Chemicals insoluble in water may be dissolved in appropriate vehicles (e.g. corn oil). If a true solution cannot be obtained, the test material may be prepared as a suspension by homogenisation in water or corn oil or in a suspending agent such as methylcellulose in water. Normally, freshly prepared solutions or suspensions of the test substance should be employed.

3.2.3 Controls

Negative controls comprise treatments of animals with an equivalent volume of the vehicle for the test compound. The positive control treatments should be *in vivo* dosage with compounds of known activity in this assay. Additional chemical class positive controls may be used where appropriate. *In vitro* application of positive control substances to hepatocyte cultures derived from negative control or test-compound treated animals (Butterworth *et al.*, 1987) is an inadequate method of validating the assay. This procedure would not control the animal treatment phases of the assay and differences in protocol and timing of operations on *in vitro*-treated cultures prevent an exact reproduction of the processing of hepatocytes taken from test compound-treated animals. In instances where experiments with two different sampling times are treated concurrently, then the *in vivo* positive control at one of the time points is sufficient to validate the whole procedure.

Positive control treatments should be at a level which gives clear increase in UDS activity. Suitable compounds are N,N'-dimethyl hydrazine dihydro-chloride (20 mg/kg) or N-nitrosodimethylamine (NDMA, 10 mg/kg) for early (4 h or less) sampling times. Unlike NDMA, which is a volatile liquid, N,N'-dimethyl hydrazine dihydrochloride is a solid so it is easier to formulate safely. At later sampling times, i.e. 12 hours or more, 2-acetylaminofluorene (2-AAF, 25 or 50 mg/kg) is a suitable positive control. For dosing many laboratories prepare 2-AAF as a suspension in corn oil. Particular care is required to ensure that this compound is well dispersed, e.g. by use of high speed homogenisation or sonication (Ashby, 1987).

3.3 ASSAY PROCEDURE
3.3.1 Study design

For *in vivo* bone marrow clastogenicity assays scoring of a single dose level, provided it is a limit dose or MTD, is considered sufficient as a screening test (Richold *et al.*, 1990). In contrast, with the rat liver UDS assay test compound data are normally obtained from at least two dose levels, as there are instances where the peak UDS response is at a dose level below the

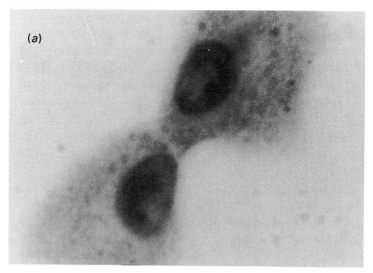

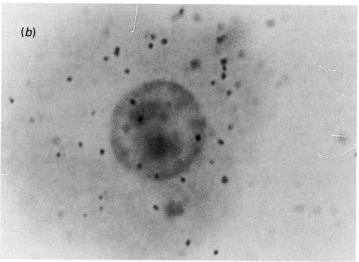

Fig. 3.1. Typical autoradiographs of hepatocytes from *in vivo* treated rats. Hepatocyte preparations are stained sufficiently to enable the operator to discern the presence of the nucleus and cytoplasm, and so ensure that cells of normal appearance and morphology are scored. Cells of abnormal shape or with pyknotic nuclei (*a*) are not scored. Deep staining of structures such as the nucleolus is to be avoided as an image analyser may then score them along with the emulsion silver grains. Consequently, in most UDS autoradiographs, the essential delineation of the cytoplasm is difficult to record photographically. In negative controls, the majority of cells will have a higher density of silver grains over the cytoplasm compared with the nucleus (*b*).

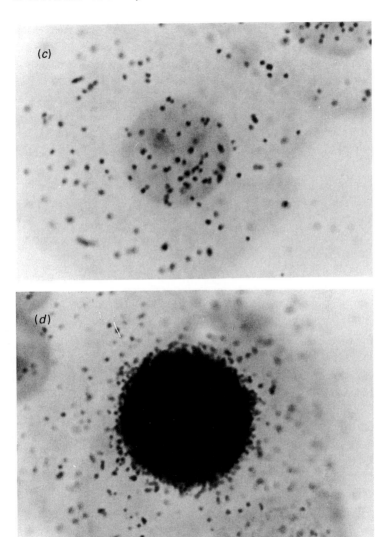

Fig. 3.1. (*cont.*).Typical autoradiographs of hepatocytes from *in vivo* treated rats. Cells in repair show a clear excess of number of silver grains over the nucleus compared with the cytoplasm (*c*). In autoradiographs, cells in S phase are readily distinguishable by their heavily blackened nuclei (*d*).

limit treatment, e.g. for technical grade dinitrotoluene (Mirsalis & Butterworth, 1982; Ashby *et al.*, 1985*b*). Additional dose levels may be included to safeguard against the possibility of the highest doses proving cytotoxic and so unscorable.

Four or five animals are treated at each dose level to permit observation of the usual level of inter-animal variation in this assay. To ensure a manageable number of animals, the experiment may be split into two parts conducted at different times. Concurrent negative and positive controls are included in each part of the experiment. In laboratories where a large historical control database has been accumulated, 1–2 negative and positive control animals have been considered sufficient to validate each part test. However, should statistical analysis of the data be desired, the negative control group for the whole experiment should have a total of at least five animals.

Hepatocytes are prepared at a single time, 12–16 hours after dosage. The investigator should consider the practicalities of achieving a consistent exposure time, e.g. by staggering the animal dose times at intervals equal to the time taken to prepare each carcass for perfusion.

The majority of compounds active in this assay produce a peak of UDS activity 12–16 hours post-treatment, however rapidly absorbed materials, e.g. the water soluble nitrosamines, have activity maxima at earlier time points. In most cases, unless there is a clear positive response at 12–16 hours, a second experiment should be conducted with a sampling time within 2–4 hours after treatment.

3.3.2   Selection of test dose levels

Test compounds should be assayed up to a maximum tolerated dose (MTD) or a dose causing cytotoxic effects in the derived hepatocyte cultures. It is recommended that non-toxic substances be assayed at a limit dose of 2000 mg/kg as applies for acute oral toxicity tests (OECD, 1987). Although the ASTM guidelines suggested a limit dose of 500 to 1000 mg/kg (Butterworth *et al.*, 1987), some carcinogens, e.g. Butter Yellow may only show clear activity when tested at more than 1000 mg/kg (Ashby & Keen, 1985).

The highest dose is usually set in an initial toxicity sighting experiment. Van den Heuval *et al.* (1990) described a fixed dose procedure whereby the MTD for a compound could be estimated by observation of signs of significant toxicity rather than lethality in dosed animals. The principles of this method have to be adapted for dose setting in *in vivo* genotoxicity assays including rat liver UDS (Mackay & Elliott, 1992). A joint party of UKEMS and the British Toxicology Society (Fielder *et al.*, 1992) have examined data for the mouse micronucleus test, as this had the largest database, and concluded that the setting of the highest test dose level based on evident toxicity rather than lethality would not adversely affect the sensitivity of the test system:

Having defined the highest test dose, subsidiary dose level(s) are set, usually spaced at approximately two- to three-fold intervals.

3.3.3 Dosing of animals

Dosing of animals is via the oral route in almost all cases, although in particular instances other routes, e.g. intravenous or inhalation may be considered more appropriate. It should be noted, however, that development of protocols for this assay has been almost exclusively with orally dosed compounds. There have been few reports of liver UDS following inhalation exposure (Doolittle *et al.*, 1984; Vincent, Theall Acre & Sarif, 1986; Working *et al.*, 1986; Trueman & Ashby, 1987). If an inhalation experiment is considered, it should be noted that parameters such as duration of dose, limit dose and sampling times have not been standardised. Similarly, with a single intravenous dose it is unlikely that the same sampling times used for oral dose experiments will be optimal. Given the location of the liver within the peritoneal cavity, dosage of test agent by intraperitoneal injection is not recommended. Young adult male rats (e.g. for Alderley Park rats, 6–9 weeks, approximately 200–250 g) are usually preferred.

3.3.4 Isolation of hepatocytes

There are various procedures to isolate hepatocytes from the treated animals. No particular advantage applies to a single method, it is for the individual laboratory to demonstrate that their isolation procedures consistently produce hepatocyte preparations with high viability.

Most laboratories use a two stage *in situ* perfusion, e.g. that described by Mitchell, Bridges & Elcombe (1984), which is modified from Rao *et al.* (1976) and Seglen (1973). A cannula is introduced into the hepatic portal vein of anaesthetised animals, and another cannula into the superior vena cava. An alternative to *in situ* perfusion is the wedge method (Lawrence, Foster & Benford, 1991). Here only the median lobe is removed from the animal and perfused via its cut surface using a needle. This enables simultaneous perfusion of, e.g. six samples with one pump so increases efficiency.

Calcium is removed by flushing with calcium-free buffer, possibly including a chelating agent such as EDTA or EGTA. During the second stage of perfusion, buffer containing calcium and collagenase or collagenase/hyaluronidase is used to dissociate the liver into single cells. Generally, the efficacy of the enzyme preparation used is batch dependent, so it is essential that batches are assayed before use. If a programme of UDS assays is being conducted, it is advisable to have as large a batch as possible in reserve.

The liver is removed from the animal, the capsule opened and the cell suspension diluted with an appropriate complete medium, e.g. Williams' or

Lebovitz L15 medium supplemented with fetal bovine serum and antibiotics (WE-complete or L15-complete). Hepatocytes are harvested by filtration and centrifugation. Samples of the suspension are taken for determination of viability by trypan blue exclusion. In the absence of compound-related cytotoxicity, mean viability values of about 75% have been reported (Ashby *et al.*, 1985*a*). The viability of the cultures is not an absolute determinant of the validity of the experiment, subsequent attachment and washing stages tend to remove non-viable cells. The results with negative and positive control animals appear to be largely independent of the initial viability of the cultures.

Cell suspensions are adjusted with complete medium to a concentration of approximately 1.5×10^5 viable cells/ml and approximately 3 ml added to 30 mm dishes or multiwell plates with 25 mm plastic tissue culture coverslips. Cultures are incubated at 37 °C for between 90 min and 2 h to enable cell attachment. At least three replicate cultures are required from each animal, but it is advisable to prepare at least three extra replicates to be held in reserve should there be any problems during slide processing.

3.3.5   Radiolabelling of cells

After cell attachment, the medium is aspirated using aseptic technique. The hepatocytes are then washed with serum-free medium (e.g. L15-incomplete or WE-incomplete). 2 ml of incomplete medium containing 10 μCi/ml [370 kBq/ml] of [³H]thymidine (specific activity usually in the range 18–40 Ci/mmol [666–1480 GBq/mmol] but up to 80 Ci/mmol [2960 GBq/mmol] has been used) is added to each culture. Cultures are incubated for at least 3 hours (4 hours has been suggested by Ashby *et al.*, 1985*a*) at 37 °C.

Cultures are washed three times with incomplete medium containing 0.25 mM unlabelled thymidine solution. This is a 'cold chase' procedure to remove excess radiolabel from the culture. The cells are then incubated overnight with 3 ml of the same medium. The cold chase procedure coupled with the short exposure to [³H]thymidine produces hepatocyte preparations with considerably lower background labelling and less intra slide variation than typically observed with *in vitro* hepatocyte UDS assays (Ashby *et al.*, 1985*a*).

3.3.6   Fixation and autoradiography

The medium is aspirated and the coverslips washed with incomplete medium or saline. Some workers swell the hepatocytes in 1% sodium citrate (Williams *et al.*, 1982; Probst *et al.*, 1981; Lonati-Galligani *et al.*, 1983); however the advantage of this step in *in vivo* assays is unknown and is normally omitted (Ashby *et al.*, 1985*a*; Butterworth *et al.*, 1987). Cells are fixed, e.g. in freshly prepared 1:3 glacial acetic acid: absolute alcohol (v/v). Three changes of fixative are commonly used, but some workers have found a single fixation for 30 minutes adequate (Burlinson, personal communication). Cells are then washed with distilled water and coverslips dried by placing them (cell side uppermost) on the edge of the appropriate dishes within a secondary container to exclude dust. When dry, coverslips are mounted, cell side up, to microscope slides approximately 0.5 cm from the unfrosted end of the slide. Slides are left flat overnight to set, in a secondary container to exclude dust. In some protocols (Probst *et al.*, 1981) cells are stained prior to autoradiography, but in most instances this is done after development to avoid any interfering chemo-development caused by the stain.

The technique most commonly used for autoradiography is essentially that of Rogers (1979). All steps involving emulsion are performed in a darkroom. Ilford K2 emulsion may be handled under Safe Light conditions, but Kodak NTB2 should be used in total darkness. Usually three slides from each animal are processed. The remaining slides are held in reserve. Slides are dipped in molten emulsion, gelled and dried at room temperature. The slides are then sealed in exposure boxes containing a small quantity of silica gel. The boxes are stored at 4 °C for at least seven days for Kodak NTB2 (Probst *et al.*, 1981) or more usually, 14 days (Williams *et al.*, 1982). The autoradiography time used depends on the particular emulsion and the exact procedure adopted, so should be standardised in each laboratory before routine use of the assay. Slides are developed using a commercial developer (e.g. Kodak D19), washed, fixed and stained. Several staining methods may be used, provided that they produce differential staining of the nucleus and cytoplasm, without interfering with scoring of emulsion grains. These include aceto-orcein (Probst *et al.*, 1981), haematoxylin/eosin (Williams *et al.*, 1982) and methyl-green pyronin Y (Butterworth *et al.*, 1987). Slides are dehydrated and mounted with coverslips.

3.3.7 Preliminary examination of slides

In each experiment, slides are examined for evidence of overt cytotoxicity, e.g. pyknosis, reduced levels of radiolabelling, reduced cell numbers. Based on these observations, slides from control animals and usually the animals that had received the two highest non-cytotoxic test agent treatments are selected for scoring.

Using a low power objective microscope scan of the hepatocyte preparations, investigators may take the opportunity to note the incidence of cells in S phase, which are readily scored by their densely labelled nuclei. However, such observations would be only a qualitative indicator to any potential induction of cell division in liver of treated animals. The incidence of S phase cells in negative control preparations is low, of the order of 1–10/1000 cells, so scoring at least 3000 cells would be required to give an accurate estimate

(Ashby *et al.*, 1986). Furthermore, the peak of induced S phase activity generally takes place 24–48 h post-treatment, later than the time points used in UDS assays, so examination for S phase cells during UDS assays may not detect all compounds with mitogenic activity. If unequivocal evidence for stimulation of liver cell division is required, a full assay for S phase induction at appropriate time points should be conducted.

Slides are coded, for example, using a random number system, by a person other than the eventual slide analyst. The analyst will therefore be unaware of the identity of slides as they are examined.

3.3.8   Quantification of UDS

In microautoradiographs the photographic emulsion is sensitive to the emission of radioactive particles. Where an emission of a particle has occurred, chemical reaction deposits silver which is visualised as a dark particle (grain) after development. The number of grains over particular areas of the cell provide a quantitative measurement of radiolabelling.

Coded slides are scored for UDS using oil immersion microscopy. Grains may be counted by eye, but this is laborious, so most investigators use automated image analysis and record grain counts with a computer. Grains may be scored using the image analyser as individual grains or with the machine in area counting mode. In area counting, the total area occupied by grains is divided by the average area/grain to derive a grain count. The area counting method is preferred, as the automatic scoring of individual grains may under-estimate the total count, especially at high values where a group of touching or overlapping grains would not be recognised as such and be scored as a single grain.

Cells of normal morphology are picked at random, with care taken to ensure no cell is read twice and that cells from each quadrant of the coverslip are read. Cells scored should have some grains over both nucleus and cytoplasm. Cells in 'S' phase appear with heavily blackened nuclei, they are easily recognised and are not analysed nor included in the number of cells examined. For each cell the nuclear count [N] (the number of silver grains over the nucleus) is observed and the instrument refocused to obtain the cytoplasmic count [C] (the number of grains in an adjacent, nuclear-sized, area of cytoplasm). The parameter used to quantify UDS is the difference between these values, the net nuclear grain count or [N–C].

The cytoplasmic grain count may be estimated by scoring that area with apparently the highest number of grains, or by taking the highest or the mean of three independent area counts. Experience suggests that, given the relatively uniform distribution of grains over the cytoplasm, the effect of the different methods of estimation on the value obtained is minimal (Butterworth *et al.*,

1987). Harbach *et al.* (1991) compared four different methods of scoring cytoplasmic grains in *in vitro* hepatocyte UDS assays. Their conclusion also was that no selection method was clearly superior. We would therefore recommend the convenience of taking only a single cytoplasmic count when scoring *in vivo* liver UDS slides.

Reaching a recommendation for the total number of cells scored per slide and per animal has not been easy. In the original UKEMS part II guidelines a minimum of 40 cells/slide was suggested (Waters *et al.*, 1984). The ASTM guideline (Butterworth *et al.*, 1987) suggested 20–50 cells/slide, 1–3 slides per animal. In laboratories new to the technique, we recommend that 100 cells/ animal be scored to familiarise the experimenters with the variability of the assay and establish a suitable historical data base. Wherever possible, 50 cells should be scored on each of two slides. A third slide is normally only read if the total number of cells scored on the other two is less than 100. There are some indications that less than 50 cells/slide may be scored without compromising the sensitivity of the assay (Harbach *et al.*, 1990). However, a decision routinely to score less than 100 cells/animal should be justified on the basis of the accumulated database in each laboratory.

3.4   DATA PROCESSING
3.4.1   Recording of data
From the nuclear [N] and cytoplasmic [C] grain counts for each cell, the net nuclear grain counts [N–C] are calculated. These data are accumulated to provide mean [N], [C] and [N–C] per slide and per animal, together with the standard deviation (SD) or standard error (SE) for each value and the percentage of cells in repair, defined as those cells with a net nuclear grain count of at least +5. Mean [N–C] values of those cells in repair are also calculated. [N], [C], [N–C] and %R, with standard deviation, are calculated for each treatment group.

Each laboratory should establish confidence limits for historical negative control data for [N], [C] and [N–C] values (Appendix 3.1) to be able to ensure that the test system is operating normally.

3.4.2   Criteria for a valid assay
For a valid assay, slide preparations should have sufficient cells of normal morphology to enable a meaningful assessment of UDS. Good slide preparations will have 200–300 scorable hepatocytes in a low power ($\times$100 magnification) field. The coefficient of variation (standard deviation/mean) for mean [N–C] from replicate slides would be expected to be of the order of 15%.

In instances where radiolabelling of the hepatocyte preparation is very high, small changes in background grain counts could give spurious [N–C] values.

Consequently, in acceptable experiments, the mean cytoplasmic count [C] of the negative controls would be expected to be in the range of 5–25. The [N–C] value of the negative control animals should be less than zero (Ashby *et al.*, 1987; Butterworth *et al.*, 1987).

Typical negative and positive control data are shown in Table 3.1.

In established laboratories mean negative control [N–C] values in the range −6 to −2 are normal (see Table 3.1 and Margolin & Risko 1988). Should laboratories consistently obtain values outside this range using the protocol described here, they should re-examine their procedures. The evaluation of responses in the liver UDS assay assumes that background levels of UDS are of this magnitude. Within a treatment group dosed on the same day, interanimal coefficient of variation for [N–C] of the order of 20% is normal, at least for negative controls and groups with [N–C] less than zero. When groups of animals show a clear positive UDS response, the magnitude of inter-animal variability is observed to be proportionally greater (Ashby *et al.*, 1987; Gallagher *et al.*, 1991). Again, if levels of variability in excess of these values occur the evaluation procedures described in 3.4.4 below are inapplicable. Values for the positive control in each experiment should show a clear positive response. In most laboratories the level of positive control treatment is selected to give a mean [N–C] value of +5 or greater, e.g. Table 3.1.

3.4.3   Definition of a positive response

For the *in vitro* hepatocyte assay Williams (1977) suggested a clear positive response would be a net grain count of +5 with at least 20% of cells in repair. These criteria were initially adopted for the *in vivo* assay, although as more experience was accumulated, it became apparent that these were over-conservative (Mirsalis, 1988). Different methods of assessment were later proposed to provide a more sensitive analysis procedure (see Appendix 3.2).

The working party did not consider these methods fully satisfactory. The use of [N–C] = +5 was clearly unacceptable as there were instances of test compounds giving rise to clear reproducible responses in rat liver UDS assays with [N–C] between 0 and +5. Given the reliability of negative control animal [N–C], such responses are clearly biologically important and outside the expected background variation of the assay, thus it would be incorrect to describe them as 'weak' or 'equivocal'.

An animal mean [N–C] = 0 or greater is recommended as an indicator of a biologically important UDS response, based on the accumulated experience of the members of the working party and others (Butterworth *et al.*, 1987; Margolin & Risko, 1988). In considering the level of net nuclear grain count indicative of an *in vivo* rat liver UDS response, it is remarkable that all laboratories report negative control mean net nuclear grain counts of less than

Table 3.1. *Control data for* in vivo *rat liver UDS*

(a) Negative controls

Laboratory [Number of rats]	Comments	N	C	[N–C]	%R
Robens [36]	Wedge perfusion	3.9 (1.3)	6.2 (1.7)	−2.4 (1.0)	2 (2)
Glaxo [61]		5.1 (1.8)	8.6 (2.5)	−3.5 (1.3)	2 (3)
Microtest [69]	Various[a] vehicles (2–17 h)	3.6 (1.7)	6.6 (3.0)	−3.0 (2.3)	1 (3)
CTL (1) [28][b]	Corn oil (2–72 h)	7.4 (1.1)	11.4 (1.6)	−4.0 (0.9)	<1 (<1)
CTL (2) [42]	Corn oil, water (4 or 12 h)	7.3 (3.4)	11.1 (4.2)	−3.8 (1.4)	1 (1)

(b) Positive controls

Laboratory [Number of rats]	Agent: (mg/kg):time (h)	N	C	[N–C]	%R
Robens [18]	MMS: (100): 2 h	14.8 (3.0)	7.5 (1.6)	+7.3 (1.0)	70 (12)
[19]	2-AAF: (50): 16 h	19.4 (5.3)	7.7 (2.2)	+11.7 (3.4)	86 (7)
Glaxo [3]	2-AAF: (25): 16 h	19.6 (3.3)	10.1 (2.3)	+9.5 (5.7)	68 (29)
[3]	2-AAF: (50): 16 h	16.2 (6.8)	9.7 (3.4)	+6.8 (3.7)	53 (23)
[13]	2-AAF: (75): 16 h	20.8 (7.4)	9.6 (2.1)	+11.2 (6.4)	72 (23)
[6]	2-AAF: (100): 16 h	27.9 (8.2)	11.6 (3.6)	+16.4 (6.0)	86 (13)
Microtest [35]	NDMA: (10): 2–6 h	19.4 (6.5)	5.0 (1.7)	+14.4 (5.6)	87 (15)
[35]	2-AAF: (50): 12–17 h	21.0 (9.0)	6.8 (3.0)	+14.3 (8.6)	88 (15)
CTL (1)[b] [6]	NDMA: (10): 2 h	29.6 (8.2)	11.5 (2.8)	+18.1 (6.5)	76 (7)
[2]	6BT: (40): 4 h	17.4	14.3	+3.2	37
[4]	6BT: (40): 12 h	32.7 (13.0)	12.1 (3.0)	+20.6 (10.2)	94 (4)
[7]	2-AAF: (10): 12 h	17.5 (2.8)	10.3 (1.0)	+7.3 (2.4)	64 (13)
[6]	2-AAF: (25): 12 h	39.0 (9.1)	16.1 (2.9)	+22.9 (8.6)	96 (5)
CTL (2) [38]	NDMA: (10): 4 h	37.3 (13.9)	11.6 (3.7)	+25.7 (11.2)	84 (11)
[41]	6BT: (40): 12 h	39.4 (17.0)	14.2 (5.1)	+25.2 (5.1)	89 (8)

N = mean animal nuclear grain count.   } Values are shown
C = mean animal cytoplasmic count.   } with standard
[N–C] = mean animal net nuclear grain count.   } deviation in
%R = % cells in repair, i.e. with [N–C] at least +5.   } parenthesis.

[a] = corn oil, water, carboxymethylcellulose, methyl cellulose, glucose solution, PBS or 0.001 M HCl.

[b] = Data obtained in experiments following those in Ashby *et al.* (1987).

6BT = 6-p-dimethylaminophenylazobenzthiazole.

zero. In Butterworth *et al.* (1987) a survey of four laboratories sampling over 200 animals gave no negative control treatment with an [N–C] value of greater than zero. Similarly, the negative control values shown in Table 3.1 are all clearly less than zero. In a statistical analysis of negative control *in vivo* UDS data produced at one laboratory during 1989–1990 the probability of obtaining a negative animal control with an [N–C] value greater than zero was determined as approximately 0.003 (Kennelly, unpublished observations).

It appears, therefore, that a mean animal [N–C] value of greater than zero represents a biologically significant departure from normal. Furthermore, in such cases, the radiolabelling of the nucleus exceeds that of the cytoplasm, so there is confidence that a real net synthesis of nuclear DNA has occurred.

The choice of [N–C] equal to zero as the criterion for positivity complements at least one of the earlier criteria of Williams (1977), in that at this mean [N–C] level the percentage of cells in repair (defined as cells with [N–C] of at least +5) is usually greater than 20%. Examination of the percentage of cells in repair is useful in that it provides a check that any increase in labelling is general, and that increased [N–C] values are not the result of a few highly labelled cells

It is therefore recommended that, under normal assay conditions, *the occurrence of a [N–C] value of zero or above in any treated animal should be taken as indicative of a UDS response.* If such an effect is reproduced then this is taken as a clear positive response in this assay.

This approach is empirical and assumes that the negative control values and interanimal variation described in Section 3.4.2 are typical. The potential weaknesses arising from the use of a single threshold value for data analysis have been noted (Margolin & Risko, 1988). However, the level chosen was based on a response considered to be biologically important and in accordance with experience of the behaviour of the test system over time in several laboratories. Too few experiments within the available UDS database had been conducted to designs which permit a rigorous retrospective evaluation of potential statistical methods, so it was decided not to recommend any particular statistical evaluation in the absence of any practical experience of its value.

3.4.4   Recommended evaluation procedure

In recommending an assessment procedure, it is assumed that laboratories new to this technique will generally obtain mean negative control animal [N–C] values in the range −6 to −2 net grains. Some laboratories might routinely observe mean negative control values outside this range, e.g. Mirsalis and coworkers have reported some negative control [N–C] values of −10 (Mirsalis *et al.*, 1988; Margolin & Risko, 1988). In such cases, the assessment criteria described below may be inapplicable. Similarly, if a laboratory is considering introducing major procedural modifications which markedly affect negative control [N–C] values (e.g. using reduced autoradiography development times) then the consequences for data evaluation should be considered. In such instances, any improvements would need to be judged against the requirement to accumulate an extensive in-house database.

Each experimental data set should be examined to observe whether negative control and test compound treated animals are within appropriate levels, e.g. 98% confidence limits of the historical database (one-sided for [N] and [N–C], two-sided for values of [C]). Normally increases in mean animal [N–C] values are indicative of a UDS response. However, any increase in mean net nuclear grain count should be the result of a real increase in nuclear labelling [N], and not be due to a depressed cytoplasm count [C]. Increased [N–C] values that do not result from increased nuclear thymidine uptake cannot be ascribed to DNA repair.

In experiments where all test compound treated animals have [N–C] values within the defined historical control limits, then the result of the assay is a clear negative.

Provided that the concurrent negative control value is within the set confidence limits, a [N–C] value of zero or greater in more than one treated animal is sufficient to assign a compound as unequivocally positive in this assay.

Applying these criteria, it is expected that the evaluation of the outcome of almost all *in vivo* rat liver UDS experiments may be made by inspection.

There may be experimental outcomes which are not readily interpreted; for example, when the negative control is within the historical range, but animals within a treatment group give increased mean net nuclear grain counts exceeding the historical range, yet below zero. There is as yet insufficient data to decide the biological importance of such an observation. Given the weight placed on any outcome of *in vivo* genotoxicity tests, we would recommend that resolution should be by repeat experiments with altered parameters, e.g. of test doses or sampling time in order to maximise any perceived test compound activity. Similarly, when the negative control value is outside the upper or lower historical negative control values any differences between treated and control animals may be difficult to evaluate. Again, the method of choice for resolution would be to conduct further experiments.

3.5 DISCUSSION

The *in vivo* liver UDS assay provides valuable data for assessment of *in vivo* genotoxic hazard which makes the necessary input of time and resources worthwhile. Before using this technique as a routine method, a laboratory should ensure that facilities are available to process sufficient animals in a single session to enable experiments of adequate size to be conducted. Preliminary experiments should be initiated to accumulate a control database: Margolin and Risko (1988) recommend a minimum of 15 negative and positive control animals. This is of particular importance as acceptability of the experiment and assessment of any test compound induced effects are by comparison with accumulated historical data.

Autoradiographs of UDS preparations are readily quantified and recorded automatically by instruments currently available. Those intending to use *in vivo* liver UDS frequently as part of a routine testing programme are advised to obtain suitable computer/image analyser equipment for slide analysis and data handling to enable an efficient throughput of studies.

APPENDIX 3.1
ANALYSIS OF *IN VIVO* RAT LIVER UDS DATA: DETERMINATION OF NEGATIVE CONTROL CONFIDENCE LIMITS

For the initial evaluation of *in vivo* rat liver UDS data, confidence limits should be placed on the historical data for mean nuclear grain counts [N], mean cytoplasmic grain counts [C] and mean net nuclear grain counts [N–C]). Limits are calculated both for groups of negative control animals and for individual animal values. The group means of negative control animals tend toward normality even though the individual animal values may not be normally distributed (Margolin & Risko, 1988), so confidence limits for group means can be readily calculated by applying normal distribution statistics. Should group mean values show a positive skew, then a square root transformation may provide a more normal distribution

For individual negative control animals, where sufficient datapoints are available, the method of choice for setting confidence limits for historical negative control values would be the normal scores method (Mitchell *et al.*, 1990) as described by Bradley (1968). To set 95% confidence limits would require data from at least 25 animals, 98 and 99% confidence limits would require at least 62 or greater than 80 animals respectively. The setting of 98% confidence limits is recommended, which would give a 1% chance of an animal exceeding the upper limit.

Where insufficient data exist for the setting of confidence limits using normal scores, limits may be calculated using a square root or arcsine transformation to obtain a normally distributed data set. Where negative values are always found, i.e. with [N–C] values, these should be multiplied by -1 prior to transformation. Using the transformed data, confidence limits may be calculated.

Once sufficient datapoints have been accrued, for example, to calculate confidence limits by the normal scores method, it is recommended that the database be updated appropriately for each new study. Data from a suitable period prior to the current study should be used to generate the confidence limits for analysis of results. The time frame/number of experiments chosen will depend on the circumstances of the individual laboratory. The number of experiments examined should enable, wherever possible, the monitoring of any drift in performance of the assay. If the negative control values for a particular experiment exceed the established historical control limits, that experiment should be examined to see whether there was any unusual factor which would disqualify the data from inclusion into the historical database. Should there be any permanent and significant change in performance, for example due to procedural modifications, it would be necessary to start the accumulation of a new historical data set.

Using these databases, comparisons may be made for both group means and individual animals with historical values. Note that individual animals should not be assessed against the group means database. The single responder (outlier) animal may present considerable problems of interpretation (Mitchell, Carlton & Gilbert, 1988) but these should not be ignored.

APPENDIX 3.2
REVIEW OF DATA ASSESSMENT METHODS

The Williams criteria for a clear positive response (Williams, 1977) were based on the distribution of individual *cell* [N–C] values within the population of negative control hepatocytes in *in vitro* studies. Cells with [N–C] values of +5 or more occur at less than 5% frequency in negative controls, so a slide showing a mean value of +5 is clearly outside the expected distribution. A clear positive was ascribed when a treatment gave rise to a mean net nuclear grain count of +5 or more with at least 20% of the cell population in repair (a cell in repair defined as one with [N–C] of +5 or more).

As the *in vivo* version of the assay was developed the Williams criteria were applied to results. There is no sound base for the direct application of these cell-based observations for the comparison of the mean [N–C] values of groups of animals in the *in vivo* assay; *in vivo* the within slide variation is smaller, but there is an added major component of interanimal variation. The experimental design of the *in vivo* assay is essentially different from that of the *in vitro* test. *In vitro* there is a comparison of the different treatments of samples drawn from the same hepatocyte population. *In vivo* the hepatocytes examined are separate primary cultures from animals receiving various pre-treatments. In practice, the use of *in vitro* analysis procedures with the *in vivo* assay has proved overconservative (Mirsalis, 1988). A mean animal [N–C] value of +5 would be highly statistically significant if compared with normal negative control [N–C] values of less than zero and, if applied stringently, would lead to false negative assignments. From consideration of historical data, Ashby *et al.* (1985) were unable to rationalise the choice of +5 net grains as the criterion for a positive response in the *in vivo* assay. Pending resolution of this uncertainty, they suggested that data evaluation would be improved if a temporary compromise criterion of +3 was operated. The problems arising from applying the Williams criteria to *in vivo* assays were also recognised by Butterworth *et al.* (1987) in formulating the ASTM guideline. In that document a compromise acceptable to all of the review groups was agreed as follows: in addition to retaining a mean net nuclear grain count of more than +5 as a clear positive, it was suggested that increased [N–C] values of between 0 and +5 could be considered a marginal response and assessed as positive if complemented by increases in the number of cells in repair and adose–response relationship.

An alternative approach was to make a statistical comparison of treated animals or groups with the concurrent negative control. However, there are currently no agreed statistical criteria. Many of the statistical tests used in hepatocyte UDS assays were designed for evaluating *in vitro* data, so might not be directly relevant to *in vivo* assays. For *in vitro* studies Casciano and Gaylor (1983) suggested an increase of three net grains over the concurrent negative control value was indicative of UDS induction. Probst and Hill (1985) set a positive as a treatment that exceeded the solvent control by three times the standard deviation of the concurrent negative control. Von der Hude, Matelblowski & Basler (1990) used a criterion for positivity of the treated culture having an [N–C] value of twice the standard deviation of the concurrent negative control value. By this criterion, even test cultures with [N–C] values well in excess of +5 can be scored as negative even with the solvent control below zero. Such methods are inappropriate for *in vivo* rat liver UDS, as they take no account of animal variability.

Comparison of treated group mean [N–C] values with that of the concurrent negative control is difficult for many reported *in vivo* UDS studies. In many experiments, there was only a single concurrent negative control animal, so there will have been no estimate of *interanimal* negative control variation. The variation due to interanimal response is considerably higher than the error in determining individual animal [N–C] values, so any analysis method that omits this factor will be oversensitive. Margolin and Risko (1988) estimated the statistical significance of the difference between the negative control and test animals using an approximation of the variance of [N–C], based on pooled historical negative control data. This analysis assumed that day-to-day variation of the negative controls was small compared with the general inter-animal variation, so that the historical database comprising essentially single animal observations over time would be a good estimate of total variation. The authors noted however, that the analysis should be reappraised if the day-to-day variation of the assay did indeed prove greater than interanimal variation.

There are, however, insufficient data from UDS studies to experimental designs that permit the satisfactory evaluation of significance testing methods. Ideally any statistical method should use the animal as the unit of analysis as this is observed to be the major component of total assay variation (Margolin & Risko, 1988; Kennelly & Greenwood, 1992). With any method, the question of statistical significance as against biological importance would need to be addressed, together with a study design which permits using the minimum number of test animals commensurate with effective detection of a UDS response. As there were insufficient data to demonstrate an effective method for data analysis, the working party decided to use in the meantime a criterion of biological significance to define a positive response.

3.6   REFERENCES

Ashby, J. (1983). The unique role of rodents in detection of possible carcinogens and mutagens. *Mutation Research*, **115**, 117–213.

Ashby, J. (1986). The prospects for a simplified and internationally harmonized approach to the detection of possible human carcinogens and mutagens. *Mutagenesis*, **1**, 3–16.

Ashby, J. (1987). The efficient preparation of corn oil suspensions. *Mutation Research*, **187**, 45.

Ashby, J., Burlinson, B. & Lefevre, P. A. (1988). Activity of 2-acetyl amino-fluorence and 4-acetylaminofluorene in an *in vitro* and an *in vivo/in vitro* assay for unscheduled DNA synthesis in the rat liver. In *Evaluation of Short-Term Tests for Carcinogenesis*, vol. 1, eds. J. Ashby, F. J. de Serres, M. D. Shelby, B. H. Margolin and G. C. Becking, Cambridge University Press, Cambridge, pp. 358–60.

Ashby, J. & Keen, W. (1985). The activity of CDA DAB and 6BT in the *in vivo* rat hepatocyte DNA repair assay. In *Comparative Genetic Toxicology: The Second UKEMS Collaborative Study*, eds. J. M. Parry and C. F. Arlett, Macmillan, London, pp. 405–10.

Ashby, J., Lefevre, P. A., Burlinson, B. & Penman, M. G. (1985*a*). An assessment of the *in vivo* rat hepatocyte DNA Repair Assay. *Mutation Research*, **156**, 1–18.

Ashby, J., Lefevre, P. A., Burlinson, B. & Penman, M. G. (1985*b*). Non-genotoxicity of 2,4,6-trinitrotoluene (TNT) to the mouse bone marrow and to the rat liver: implications for its carcinogenicity. *Archives of Toxicology*, **58**, 14–19.

Ashby, J., Lefevre, P. A., Burlinson, B. & Beije, B. (1986). Potent mitogenic activity of 4-acetylaminofluorene to the rat liver. *Mutation Research*, **172**, 271–9.

Ashby, J., Trueman, R. W., Mohammed, R. & Barber, G. (1987). Positive and negative control observations for the *in vivo* rat liver assay for unscheduled DNA synthesis (UDS). *Mutagenesis,* **2** (6), 489–90.

Bermudez, E., Tillery, D. & Butterworth, B. E. (1979). The effect of 2,4-diaminotoluene and isomers of dinitrotoluene on unscheduled DNA synthesis in primary rat hepatocytes. *Environmental Mutations,* **1,** 391–8.

Bradley, J. V. (1968). Normal scores tests. In *Distribution-Free Statistical Tests,* Prentice-Hall, Englewood Cliffs, NJ, pp. 146–63.

Butterworth, B. E., Ashby, J., Bermudez, E., Casciano, D., Mirsalis, J., Probst, G. & Williams, G. M. (1987). A protocol and guide for *in vivo* rat hepatocyte DNA repair assay. *Mutation Research,* **189,** 123-33.

Campbell, R. C. (1974). Comparing several samples. In *Statistics for Biologists,* 2nd edn, Cambridge University Press, Cambridge, pp. 50–76.

Casciano, D. A. & Gaylor, D. W. (1983). Statistical criteria for evaluating chemicals as positive or negative in the hepatocyte/DNA repair assay. *Mutation Research,* **122,** 81–6.

Cleaver, J. E. & Thomas, G. H. (1981). Measurement of unscheduled DNA synthesis by autoradiography. In *DNA Repair, A Laboratory Manual of Research Procedures,* eds. E. C. Friedberg and P. C. Hanawalt, Marcel Dekker, New York, pp. 277–87.

Department of Health (1989). Report on health and social subjects, *35 Guidelines for the Testing of Chemicals for Mutagenicity.* HMSO, London.

Djordjevic, B. & Tolmach, L. J. (1967). Responses of synchronous populations of Hela cells to ultra violet irradiation at selected stages of the generation cycle. *Radiation Research,* **32,** 327–46.

Doolittle, D. J., Bermudez E., Working, P. K. & Butterworth, B. E. (1984). Measurement of genotoxic activity in multiple tissues following inhalation exposure to dimethylnitrosamine. *Mutation Research,* **141,** 123–7.

Fielder, R. J., Allen, J., Boobis, A., Botham, P., Doe, J., Esdale, D., Gatehouse, D., Hodgson-Walker G., Morton, D., Kirkland, D. & Richold, M. (1992). Report of the BTS/UKEMS working group on dose setting in *in vivo* mutagenicity assays. *Mutagenesis* **7,** 313–16.

Fox, M. (1988). The case for retention of mammalian cell mutagenicity assays. *Mutagenesis,* **3,** 459–61.

Furihata, C. & Matsushima, T. (1987). Use of *in vivo/in vitro* unscheduled DNA synthesis for identification of organ-specific carcinogens. *CRC Critical Reviews in Toxicology,* **17,** 245–77.

Gallagher, J. E., Shank, T., Lewtas, J., Lefevre, P. A. & Ashby, J. (1991). Relative sensitivities of ^{32}P-postlabelling and the autoradiographic UDS assay in the liver of rats exposed to 2-acetylaminofluorene (2AAF). *Mutation Research,* **25,** 247–57.

Glauert, H. P., Kennan, W. S., Sattler, G. L. & Pitot, H. C. (1985). Assays to measure the induction of unscheduled DNA in cultured hepatocytes. In *Progress in Mutation Research,* vol. 5, eds. J. Ashby, F. J. de Serres, M. Draper, M. Ishidate, B. H. Margolin, B. E. Matter and M. D. Shelby, Elsevier Scientific Publishers, Amsterdam, pp. 371–5.

Hanawalt, P. C., Cooper, P. K., Ganesan, A. K. & Smith, C. A. (1979). DNA repair in bacteria and mammalian cells. *Annual Reviews in Biochemistry,* **48,** 783–836.

Harbach, P. R., Rostami, H. J., Aaron, C. S., Wiser, S. K. & Grzegorczyk, C. R. (1990). Statistical evaluation of the number of cells scored in the rat primary hepatocyte unscheduled DNA synthesis (UDS) assay. *Environmental Mutagen Society Meeting*, Alberquerque, USA, Abstract 84.

Harbach, P. R., Rostami, H. J., Aaron, C. S., Wiser, S. K. & Grzegorczyk, C. R. (1991). Evaluation of four methods for scoring cytoplasmic grains in the *in vitro* unscheduled DNA synthesis (UDS) assay. *Mutation Research*, **252**, 139–48.

Joachim, F. & Decad, G. M. (1984). Induction of unscheduled DNA synthesis in primary rat hepatocytes by benzidine-congener derived azo dyes in the *in vitro* and *in vivo* assays. *Mutation Research*, **136**, 147–52.

Kennelly, J. C. & Greenwood, M. R. (1992). The effect of reducing the number of cells scored on the performance of the *in vivo* rat liver UDS assay. *Mutagenesis* **7**, 381–2.

Lawrence, J. N., Foster, B. & Benford D. J. (1991). The application of a wedge perfusion technique to the *in vivo–in vitro* rat hepatocyte DNA repair assay. *Mutation Research*, **252**, 129–37.

Lonati-Galligani, M., Lohman, P. H. M. & Berends, F. (1983). The validity of the autoradiographic method for detecting DNA repair synthesis in rat hepatocyte primary culture. *Mutation Research*, **113**, 145–60.

Mackay, J. M. & Elliott, B. M. (1992). Dose-ranging and dose-setting for *in vivo* genetic toxicology studies. *Mutation Research*, **271**, 97–9.

Margolin, B. H. & Risko, K. J. (1988). The statistical analysis of *in vivo* genotoxicity data: case studies of the rat hepatocyte UDS and mouse bone marrow micronucleus assays. In *Evaluation of Short-term Tests for Carcinogenesis*, vol. 1, eds. J. Ashby, F. J. de Serres, M. D. Shelby, B. H. Margolin and G. C. Becking, Cambridge University Press, Cambridge, pp. 29–43.

Martin, C. N., McDermid, A. C. & Garner, R. C. (1978). Testing of known carcinogens and non-carcinogens for the ability to induce unscheduled DNA synthesis in HeLa cells. *Cancer Research*, **38**, 2621–7.

Mirsalis, J. C. (1988). Summary report on the performance of the *in vivo* DNA repair assays. In *Evaluation of Short-term Tests for Carcinogenesis*, vol. 1, eds. J. Ashby, F. J. de Serres, M. D. Shelby, B. H. Margolin and G. C. Becking, Cambridge University Press, Cambridge, pp. 345–57.

Mirsalis, J. C. & Butterworth B. E. (1980). Detection of unscheduled DNA synthesis in hepatocytes isolated from rats treated with genotoxic agents: an *in vivo* and *in vitro* assay for potential carcinogens and mutagens. *Carcinogenesis*, **1**, 621–5.

Mirsalis, J. C. & Butterworth, B. E. (1982). Induction of unscheduled DNA synthesis in rat hepatocytes following *in vivo* treatment with dinitrotoluene. *Carcinogenesis*, **3**, 241–5.

Mirsalis, J. C., Tyson, C. K. & Butterworth, B. E. (1982). Detection of genotoxic carcinogens in the *in vivo/in vitro* hepatocyte DNA repair assay. *Environmental Mutagenesis*, **4**, 553–62.

Miraslis, J. C., Tyson, C. K., Loh, E. K. N., Bakke, J. B., Ramsey, M. J., Hamilton, C. M. & Steinmetz, K. L. (1988). An evaluation of the ability of benzo(a)pyrene, pyrene, 2- and 4-acetylaminofluorene to induce unscheduled DNA synthesis and cell proliferation in the livers of male rats and mice treated *in vivo*.In *Evaluation of Short-term Tests for Carcinogenesis*, vol. 1, eds. J. Ashby, F. J. de Serres, M. D. Shelby, B. H. Margolin and G. C. Becking, Cambridge University Press, Cambridge, pp. 361–6.

Mitchell, A. M., Bridges, J. W. & Elcombe, C. R. (1984). Factors influencing peroxisome proliferation in cultured rat hepatocytes. *Archives in Toxicology*, **55**, 239–46.

Mitchell, I. deG. (1987). The interaction of statistical significance, biology of dose-response and test design in the assessment of genotoxicity data. *Mutagenesis*, **2**, 141–5.

Mitchell, I. deG., Carlton, J. B. & Gilbert, P. J. (1988). The detection and importance of outliers in the *in vivo* micronucleus assay. *Mutagenesis*, **3**, 491–5.

Mitchell, I. deG., Rees, R. W., Gilbert, P. J. & Carlton, J. B. (1990). The use of historical data for identifying biologically unimportant but statistically significant results in genotoxicity tests. *Mutagenesis*, **5**, 159–64.

OECD (1987). *OECD Guidelines for Testing of Chemicals: 401 Acute Oral Toxicity*, Organisation for Economic Co-operation and Development, Paris.

Probst, G. S. & Hill, L. E. (1985). Tests for the induction of unscheduled DNA synthesis in cultured hepatocytes. In *Progress in Mutation Research*, vol. 5, eds. J. Ashby, F. J. de Serres, M. Draper, M. Ishidate, B. H. Margolin, B. E. Matter and M. D. Shelby, Elsevier Scientific Publishers, Amsterdam, pp. 381–6.

Probst, G. S., McMahon, E., Hill, L. E., Thompson, Z., Epp, J. K. & Neal, S. B. (1981). Chemically induced unscheduled DNA synthesis in primary cultures of adult rat hepatocytes: a comparison with bacterial mutagenicity using 218 compounds. *Environmental Mutagenesis*, **3**, 11–32.

Puri, E. C. & Müller, D. (1989). Testing of hydralazine in *in vivo–in vitro* hepatocyte assays for UDS and stimulation of replicative DNA synthesis. *Mutation Research*, **218**, 13–19.

Rao, M. L., Rao, G. S., Holler, M., Breuer, H., Schattenberg, P. J. & Stein, W. D. (1976). Uptake of cortisol by isolated rat liver cells. A phenomenon indicative of carrier mediation and simple diffusion. *Hoppe Zeylers Zeitschrift Physiologische Chemie*, **357**, 573–84.

Rasmusson, R. E. & Painter, R. B. (1964). Evidence for repair of ultra violet damaged deoxyribonucleic acid in cultured mammalian cells. *Nature*, **203**, 1360–2.

Regan, J. D. & Setlow, R. B. (1974). Two forms of repair in the DNA of human cells damaged by chemical carcinogens and mutagens. *Cancer Research*, **34**, 3318–25.

Reitz, R. H., Watanabe, P. G., McKenna, M. J. & Gehring, P. J. (1980). Effects of vinylidine chloride on DNA synthesis and DNA repair in the rat and mouse: a comparative study with dimethylnitrosamine. *Toxicology and Applied Pharmacology*, **52**, 357–70.

Richhold, M., Ashby, J., Bootman, J., Chandley, A., Gatehouse, D. G. & Henderson, L. (1990). *In vivo* cytogenetics assays. In *Basic Mutagenicity Tests: UKEMS Recommended Procedures*, ed. D. Kirkland, Cambridge University Press, Cambridge, pp. 115–37.

Rogers, A. W. (1979). *Techniques of Autoradiography*, 3rd edn, Elsevier/North-Holland Biomedical Press, pp. 368–70.

Schmetzer, P., Pool, B. I., Lefevre, P. A., Callander, R. D., Ratpan, F., Tinwell, H. & Ashby, J. (1990). Assay-specific genotoxicity of N-nitrosodibenzylamine to the rat liver *in vivo*. *Environmental Molecular Mutagenesis*, **15**, 190–7.

Seglen, P. O. (1973). Preparation of rat liver cells. *Experimental Cell Research*, **82**, 391–8.

Stich, H. F. & Kieser (1974). Use of DNA repair synthesis in detecting organotrophic actions of chemical carcinogens. *Proceedings of the Society of Experimental Biology and Medicine*, 1229–42.

Trueman, R. W. & Ashby, J. (1987). Lack of UDS activity in the livers of mice and rats exposed to dichoromethane. *Environmental and Molecular Mutagenesis*, **10**, 189–95.

Van den Heuval, M. J., Clark, D. G., Fielder, R. J., Koundakjian, P. P., Oliver, G. J. A., Pelling, D., Tomlinson, N. J. & Walker, A. P. (1990). The international validation of a fixed dose procedure as an alternative to the classical LD_{50} test. *Food and Chemical Toxicology*, **28**, 469–82.

Vincent, D. R., Theall Acre, G. & Sarrif, A. M. (1986). Genotoxicity of 1,2-butadiene. Assessment by the unscheduled DNA synthesis assay in B6C3F1 mice and Sprague–Dawley rats *in vivo* and *in vitro*. *1986 EMS Meeting*, Abstract no. 235.

von der Hude, W., Matelblowski, R. & Basler, A. (1990). Induction of DNA synthesis in primary rat hepatocytes by epoxides. *Mutation Research*, **245**, 145–50.

Waters, R., Ashby, J., Burlinson, B., Lefevre, P., Barrett, R. & Martin, C. (1984). Unscheduled DNA synthesis. In *Report of the UKEMS Sub-committee on Guidelines for Mutagenicity Testing, Part II Supplementary Tests*, ed. B. J. Dean, United Kingdom Environmental Mutagen Society, Swansea, pp. 63–87.

Williams, G. M. (1976). Carcinogen induced DNA repair in primary rat liver cell cultures. A possible screen for chemical carcinogens. *Cancer Letters*, **1**, 231–6.

Williams, G. M. (1977). Detection of chemical carcinogens by unscheduled DNA synthesis in rat liver primary cell cultures. *Cancer Research*, **37**, 1845–51.

Williams, G. M. (1978). Further improvements in the hepatocyte primary culture DNA repair test for carcinogens: detection of biphenyl derivatives. *Cancer Letters*, **4**, 69–75.

Williams, G. M. & Laspia, M. F. (1979). The detection of various nitrosamines in the hepatocyte primary culture/DNA repair test. *Cancer Letters*, **66**, 199–206.

Williams, G. M., Laspia, M. F. & Dunkel, V. C. (1982). Reliability of the hepatocyte primary culture/DNA repair test in testing coded carcinogens and non-carcinogens. *Mutation Research*, **97**, 359–70.

Working, P. K., Doolittle, D. J., Smith-Oliver, T., White, R. D. & Butterworth, B. E. (1986). Unscheduled DNA synthesis in rat tracheal epithelial cells, hepatocytes and spermatocytes following exposure to methyl chloride *in vitro* and *in vivo*. *Mutation Research*, **162**, 219–24.

4

Measurement of covalent binding to DNA *in vivo*

C. N. Martin   P. D. Lawley
D. Phillips   S. Venitt   R. Waters

4.1   INTRODUCTION
4.1.1   Terms of reference
The members of the working party limited themselves to discussion of methods of detecting covalent DNA binding which rely on the use of radiolabelled test material. It was felt that, at the present time, the [^{32}p]-post-labelling technique is still a research tool, and that more developmental work will be required before this method can be applied to the routine screening of all types of chemicals. Nevertheless, the technique is very powerful and clearly there is great potential advantage in any technique that will allow the DNA binding ability of a compound to be investigated without recourse to the synthesis and use of a radioisotopically labelled compound. Therefore some remarks on postlabelling can be found in Appendix 4.5.

4.1.2   Principles of the assay
The object of the assay described in this chapter is to detect and to measure the formation of chemical adducts between a test compound (or its metabolites) and DNA. References on the subject are too numerous to cite; however, some selected texts are worthy of mention: Grover, 1979; Searle, 1984; Cooper & Grover, 1990.

Groups of animals are dosed with a radiolabelled chemical of known specific radioactivity and radiochemical purity. At given times after treatment, animals are killed, major organs and tissues are removed, DNA is extracted and purified and the level of radioactivity of DNA samples is determined. DNA shown to be radioactive is enzymically digested to deoxyribonucleosides. High-performance liquid chromatography (HPLC) of the digest is used to determine whether the radioactivity bound to DNA represents covalently bound adducts, metabolic incorporation (which has no genotoxic significance), or non-specific binding of unknown significance.

Covalent binding of chemicals to DNA, with the formation of chemically stable adducts, plays a major role in the mode of action of chemical mutagens and carcinogens, and is a property common to a wide variety of carcinogens (for review, see Osborne, 1984). DNA-adduct formation occurs mainly by the reaction of electrophiles with nucleophilic centres in DNA. Adducts range in size and complexity from simple alkyl groups to bulky multi-ring residues of chemicals such as polycyclic aromatic hydrocarbons, aromatic amines and aflatoxins. DNA bases are the main target of attack, the most vulnerable base being guanine.

Some genotoxic chemicals are intrinsically reactive and form adducts directly with DNA in a living cell. Other genotoxic chemicals are indirect-acting agents. Such compounds are not electrophilic *per se*, but are converted to electrophiles by cellular enzyme systems.

In the majority of cases, a single chemical will give rise to several different DNA adducts. This may be due to the production of several different metabolites from the same chemical, to reaction of a single reactive species with atoms of different nucleophilicities in the DNA molecule, or to a combination of both. Stereochemical and physicochemical constraints also play a part in determining the spectrum of DNA adducts formed by a given compound.

The formation of a DNA adduct is not of itself a mutagenic event. Rather, a DNA adduct is considered to be a pro-mutagenic lesion, i.e. a chemical modification of DNA structure which may have biological consequences, including mutation. Whether or not mutation follows adduct formation depends on the chemistry of the given adducts, and the biological response of the cells in which they occur. For example, a methyl group at N-7 of guanine is much less mutagenic than the same group at O^6 of guanine, since the latter participates in hydrogen-bond formation during complementary base-pairing, whilst the former does not. By contrast, a bulky adduct such as that formed by aflatoxin B_1 at N-7 of guanine is highly mutagenic, presumably because it causes gross distortion of the DNA structure.

The biological response to DNA adducts can be complex, involving an interaction between DNA replication, cell division and DNA repair. DNA adducts can only lead to mutation if the cell which contains the adducted DNA remains viable and produces daughter cells. Thus cellular DNA which is adducted in a way which prevents replication, for example, by inter-strand crosslinking, will not divide and mutation will not result. On the other hand, a cell whose DNA contains adducts, and which is capable of dividing, may produce mutant progeny. The type of mutation produced will depend on how the adducted DNA is processed or repaired. Some examples of repair and the consequences in terms of mutagenicity are given below:

1. The chemical residue itself, e.g. a methyl group, might be removed, either spontaneously or by enzymic dealkylation via alkyltransferase. This would leave the DNA undamaged and its coding properties intact.

2. The DNA strand which contains the adducted base may act as a template for replication, with the possibility that the adducted base may pair with the 'wrong' base. For example, O^6-methylguanine may pair with thymine instead of cytosine, resulting, in the next round of replication, in a GC to AT transition, i.e., a base-pair substitution mutation.

3. The adducted base might be lost by spontaneous hydrolysis, or removed enzymically, by a repair-glycosylase, leaving an apurinic or apyrimidinic site.

4. The adducted base might be excised by a repair-endonuclease, leaving a DNA strand break.

   Events 3. and 4. produce stretches of DNA which can act as substrates for repair enzymes; the results of repair depend on the nature of the DNA damage and the specificity of the enzyme. Error-free repair will restore the original DNA coding, whereas various forms of error-prone repair will give rise to gene mutation, chromosomal anomalies and/or cell death.

4.1.3   Relevance and limitations

4.1.3.1   *When to carry out a DNA binding assay*

When a DNA binding assay should be carried out relative to other molecular toxicological and toxicological studies is the subject of debate. The consensus of the Working Group was that the nature and cost of such studies would normally dictate that they most usefully be performed later in the progress of a test material through the battery of toxicological studies. Furthermore, this type of study would not be used routinely; rather, the requirement to carry out a DNA binding assay would be dictated by specific circumstances. An example of such circumstances might be a situation where a compound shows no indication of carcinogenicity or *in vivo* mutagenicity but evidence exists of activity in *in vitro* gene mutation assays. In these circumstances it would be unclear as to whether the *in vitro* data is suggestive of a biological effect which is missed by the relative insensitivity of *in vivo* studies; or whether, due to lack of or changes in cellular compartmentalisation, the *in vitro* data represents a false-positive result. Under these circumstances, the DNA binding assay might be employed as a sensitive *in vivo* assay providing information as to the possible pro-mutagenicity of the test material in the whole animal.

4.1.3.2 Examples of false negatives

Certain classes of mutagenic or carcinogenic chemicals may exert their effects without forming DNA adducts or without forming adducts detectable by assays using radiolabelled test material. Thus a chemical which has shown no ability to bind to DNA cannot be guaranteed to be devoid of genetic activity. For example, anti-tumour drugs, such as etoposide and teniposide, which induce DNA strand breaks by interfering with topoisomerase II (Ross, Sullivan & Chow, 1988) and are potent genotoxins in mammalian cells (Gupta *et al.*, 1987; DeMarini *et al.*, 1987) but do not bind covalently to DNA. Amsacrine is genotoxic by a similar mechanism (Andersson & Kihlman, 1989). Bleomycin, a potent clastogen, binds non-covalently to DNA, probably by intercalation and catalyses free-radical production by reduction of oxygen (Muraoka, Takita & Umazawa, 1986).

Anti-metabolites used in cancer chemotherapy block cell replication by interfering with the biochemical pathways for biosynthesis of nucleic acid precursors rather than by direct reaction with DNA (Kunz, 1988; Sowers *et al.*, 1988).

Spindle poisons (for example, the vinca alkaloids vincristine and vinblastine) represent another class of agents which induce genotoxic events indirectly and do not form DNA adducts (Degraeve, 1978; Ehling *et al.*, 1988; Rohrborn & Basler, 1981; Basler, 1986; Onfelt, 1986).

DNA damage caused by free radicals will not be detected by assays for DNA binding using radiolabelled test compounds. Free radicles may be generated by a variety of chemicals including, for example, peroxides.

4.1.3.3 Effects of adduct structure

Many of the sites in DNA bases are potentially reactive, but the relative proportions of products will be dependent on the nature of the reagents. (For more detailed reviews covering specific carcinogens, see various chapters in Searle, 1984.) The position of substitution and the stereochemistry of the resultant adduct can have a much greater genotoxic effect than the number of adducts induced. Thus, for example, methylation at the O^6 atom of guanine produces a highly pro-mutagenic adduct whereas methylation to produce N-7 methylguanine has far less significance for mutation induction (Lawley, in Searle, 1984). These differences are primarily due to the extent of interference with normal hydrogen bonding during base-pairing. As an example of differences in adduct pro-mutagenicity with more bulky carcinogens, the mutagenicity of the major adduct of benzidine (at the C-8 atom of guanine) is many times less mutagenic than the major adduct of aflatoxin (which involves substitution at the N-7 atom of guanine (Martin & Jennings, 1990). The reason for this appears to be the low steric hindrance created by the benzidine adduct.

Thus this lesion is a poor inducer of DNA repair which may be error-prone leading to mutational events. DNA binding assays can give a quantitative measure of the adducts detected but can give little insight as to their biological significance.

The level and pattern of adduct formation will be determined by absorption, distribution and metabolism, which in turn will be governed by the age, sex, strain and species of the test animal as well as the dose and route of administration of the test compound.

4.1.3.4 *Effects of extraction and DNA digestion procedures*

Adducts in DNA can be unstable and for this reason could be formed and lost before measurement can take place. Such losses can occur as a consequence of the action of biological systems such as DNA repair or as a consequence of chemical instability. The losses could occur naturally or be induced by the DNA extraction procedure. Some factors worthy of note are presented below.

Fig. 4.1(*a*) shows hydrolysis of the *N*-glycosidic linkages between 7-alkylguanine and deoxyribose in alkylated DNA which occurs at neutral pH and 37 °C at appreciable rates but is accelerated under acidic conditions. Also shown is the effect of mild alkaline conditions (e.g. pH 9) on 7-alkylguanine in DNA which can be converted into the imidazole ring-opened form. R represents the alkyl group and dR represents deoxyribose.

Prior to HPLC analysis, DNA must be hydrolysed using low pH, heat or enzymes. In view of the fact that acid hydrolysis of DNA is relatively facile, with purines being removed much more rapidly than pyrimidines, it is to be expected that alkylation of DNA, which affects mainly basic atoms, will also destabilize DNA in the same way.

Hydrolysis of *N*-glycosidic linkages between 3- or 7-alkylpurines and deoxyribose in alkylated DNA (Fig. 4.1(*a*)) occurs at neutral pH and 37 °C, at appreciable rates. Thus the half-life of 3-methyladenine is about 309 h, and 7-methylguanine about 100 h, under these conditions.

Other hydrolytic reactions can alter chemical structure of the adducts while leaving them attached to the DNA macromolecule. For example, if mild alkaline conditions, e.g. pH 9, are used during enzymic digestion of DNA, 7-alkylguanine residues would be to some extent converted into the imidazole ring-opened forms, i.e. with the basic moiety becoming a 2-amino-4-oxy-5-alkylamino-6-deoxyribosylaminopyrimidine (Fig. 4.1(*a*)). These reactions appear to be accompanied by isomerism in the affected deoxyriboside, since they yield more than a single product, with the same UV spectrum indicative of the same pyrimidine moiety.

In some instances, reactions subsequent to initial alkylation of DNA can stabilize the original product. Thus, with formaldehyde, the unstable primary hydroxymethylamino derivatives can react further to yield cross-linked bases (Fig. 4.1(*b*)) but this will represent only a relatively small part of the original products.

In order to detect, and in some cases to identify, chemical modifications of DNA, enzymic degradation through oligonucleotides, then deoxyribonucleotides, to deoxyribonucleosides, has been widely used. Methods have developed from early work on reactions of [3H]-labelled polycyclic aromatic hydrocarbons with cellular DNA (Baird & Brookes, 1973). The [3H]-labelled DNA

Fig. 4.1(*b*) shows a product of cytosine in DNA after reaction with formaldehyde; the unstable primary hydroxymethylamino derivative can then react further to yield cross-linking with adenine.

was digested with DNase (at pH7, 37°C, 4 h), venom phosphodiesterase (phosphodiesterase I, a 5'-exonuclease, at pH 9, 37 °C, 44–60 h), then alkaline phosphatase (from *Escherichia coli*, type III, at pH 9, 37 °C, 24–48 h).

Almost all chemical mutagens and carcinogens yield phosphotriester groups in DNA (which can be detected by their hydrolysis in strongly alkaline solution; 0.5 M NaOH, 37 °C, 1 h), causing strand breakage (Shooter, 1978). It may therefore be expected that these reactions would block the progress of exonuclease-mediated digestion. However, following the procedure specified, relatively slow release of methylphosphotriesters from methylated DNA appeared to be complete after about 24 h (Swenson & Lawley, 1978). The question remains, however, whether complete digestion of chemically modified DNA can be achieved in general. All reports of chromatographic analyses of digests from DNA labelled *in vivo* with [³H] from polycyclic aromatic hydrocarbons show [³H]-labelled material that elutes close to the void volume of columns and can be distinguished from the unmodified deoxyribonucleosides, which also usually incorporate [³H] to some extent. Various reasons for this have been offered, in addition to incomplete digestion of DNA, for example, cross-linking of DNA to protein, but the consensus remains that there is no single explanation (Osborne & Crosby, 1987).

Some methods use nuclease P_1 to digest DNA. It has been found that some modified deoxyribonucleotides are resistant to dephosphorylation by nuclease P_1 (an enzyme with 3'-nucleotidase activity for unmodified nucleotides) a finding which may indicate that some chemically modified nucleotides might be more resistant than the normal nucleotides to the action of other enzymes used in DNA digestion.

In conclusion, it is generally assumed that the conventional enzymic digestion of DNA, chemically modified to the relatively small extents expected *in vivo*, will normally effect virtually complete liberation of modified deoxyribonucleosides. It is further assumed that these will show retention in conventional HPLC to either about the same times as normal non-modified DNA deoxyribonucleosides, or to rather longer times. Therefore any radio-labelled material that elutes before the normal deoxyribonucleosides must be assumed not to represent adducts. Incorporation of label into the normal deoxyribonucleosides will be indicated by coincidence of radioactivity and UV absorption. Preferably, this should be checked using more than one chromatographic system. Partial losses of products such as 3- and 7-alkylpurines, that are labile to acid hydrolysis, will be expected during incubation, but these would be expected to be relatively small at pHs close to neutrality, and the products would chromatograph as alkylpurine bases rather than deoxyribonucleosides. Depurination of DNA to small extents does not appear to affect its enzymic digestion.

4.2   THE PROCEDURE
4.2.1   Prerequisites

Many of these are common to all assays for chemical genotoxic activity (see Chapter 1). However, particular note should be taken of the following:

- Solid, liquid or gaseous test chemical which must be generally labelled with [^{3}H] or, preferably, [^{14}C] to a specific activity which would allow the injection or administration of not less than 2×10^9 dpm per kg body weight.
- The same compound, unlabelled to act as standard and, in some cases, diluent of labelled material.
- Data showing the labelled compound to be identical with the unlabelled standard. The compound to be >99% pure with a radio-chemical purity of the same order.

4.2.2   Minimum requirements in design of the study
4.2.2.1   Animals

The species used should be chosen to complement any other toxico-logical studies performed. With this in mind, any appropriate mammalian species (usually rodent) may be used, e.g. rats, mice or Syrian hamsters.

At least six animals per sex per experimental and control groups should be used. All six animals per group should be treated and their organs removed and washed. It may only be necessary to process organs from three, the remainder being stored at -90 °C for possible further investigation in light of the experimental findings. It should be sufficient to examine only one sex. However both sexes should be examined if sex differences in response to the test material are suspected. If germ cells are of interest as potential targets, particular attention must be paid to the choice of sex.

Analysis of the food and water provided for the animals must be carried out and it must be demonstrated from these results that neither contain any biological or chemical entity which might interfere with the conduct of the study.

The decision whether or not to withdraw food during the treatment period will need to be made on a case-by-case basis.

Prior to, and after, the study, all cages should be washed in detergent capable of removing radioactivity, rinsed and dried before use. Cages must be checked for radioactive contamination before use and before being returned to circulation.

4.2.2.2   Test material

The test material should be prepared in an appropriate vehicle which is compatible with the solubility and the chemistry of the compound, the animal species to be treated and the route of administration.

The specific radioactivity needs to be high enough to permit doses which are not acutely toxic within the time period of the study. The compound should be generally radiolabelled to prevent possible cleavage of the radiolabelled moiety from the active centre during metabolism. To achieve the sensitivity required (at least 1 pmol of putative adduct per unit of DNA analysed) it is desirable that at least 4 mCi/kg (for [^{3}H]-labelled material) and 1.5 mCi/kg (for [^{14}C]-labelled material) of labelled test article should be administered. The doses required will therefore affect the specific activity required to achieve these radiochemical doses. Due to potential problems of tritium exchange, use of [^{14}C]-labelled material is preferred if possible.

The test material must be at least of the same chemical purity as that of the material intended for commercial use. The radiochemical purity must be greater than 90% and preferably greater than 99%.

Radiolysis of the compound must be avoided where possible. If this does occur the extent must be measured over the period of exposure. Low temperature and storage in certain solvents can reduce this (advice should be sought from the radiochemical supplier).

The route of administration of the test article would normally be related to the expected route of exposure in man but the final decision should be reviewed on a case-by-case basis.

Depending upon the metabolism of the compound, and its pharmacodynamics and pharmacokinetics, the most relevant dosing regime must be determined. The choices are a) a dose range with a fixed termination time or b) a single dose with groups terminating at different intervals after the exposure.

To use a dose range at a single time point, it must be shown beyond doubt that the time chosen gives the maximum chance of detecting putative activity with DNA. As this may prove difficult to achieve, it is recommended that activity with time be the preferred regime. In this case, actual time points will be based on the known pharmacodynamics and pharmacokinetics of the compound. A minimum of three time points should be used. Experience with a number of compounds has shown that maximal binding often occurs around 24 hours after exposure, though there are compounds which, due to factors such as effective repair, exhibit maximal binding at much earlier times. Actual times must be considered on a case-by-case basis.

Although not directly associated with measurement of DNA binding, it is recommended that most of the radioactivity administered is accounted for as far as is practicable. It is unnecessary to count the whole body, but it is desirable to determine the distribution of the radiolabel by measuring the radioactivity of samples of the major organs under investigation. The extent of excretion in urine and removal in faeces should also be measured. It may be desirable to make separate timed collections. The total of all the above figures will give a good approximation of the fate of the administered radiolabel and serve as a useful quality control measure (see Dring, 1987).

It is not mandatory to include a positive control in the study. However, any lab intending to carry out such studies should first validate the assay by using one or more radiolabelled positive control compounds. Compounds for which the quantitative DNA binding pattern in various organs has been established should be chosen. The adduct structure should also have been elucidated and the chromatographic profiles of these adducts documented in the literature.

4.2.2.3   *Organs*

The organs chosen for study will depend on the metabolism of the compound. It is prudent to remove and store, in liquid nitrogen, all major organs not investigated. The liver should almost invariably be included among the organs investigated. The list below shows the most common organs which may be exposed to the highest levels of the compound or may be of other interest, e.g. bone marrow for determining the relevance of bone marrow cytogenetic assays:

- liver
- kidneys
- lung
- stomach
- small intestine
- large intestine
- bladder
- bone marrow
- gonads

4.2.2.4   *Reagents*

Unless specified for good reason, all chemicals used should be of analytical reagent grade. Details of the formulation and preparation of reagents made at the testing laboratory must be given in the final report.

4.2.3   **Protocol**

There are numerous literature references which cite methodologies for DNA extraction and adduct quantification and analysis. Appendix 4.1

presents an example protocol as a guide to the application of these methodologies to the screening of test chemicals.

4.3   DATA PROCESSING AND PRESENTATION

4.3.1   Recording and storage of data
This is discussed in general terms in Chapter 1.

4.3.2   Appropriate statistical treatment
A formal statistical treatment of data from DNA binding assays is not required where the results of an adequately conducted experiment are decisively negative, i.e. where no radioactivity can be detected. Where low levels are detected, e.g. a doubling or less of the background, higher precision can be obtained by prolonged counting, for example, by setting the instrument to count a predetermined and large number of counts. This is better than repeating a short count many times.

Evidence of linearity of scintillation counting versus amount of DNA counted, i.e. doubling the amount added to the scintillation vial should double the number of counts recorded, is the best method for checking whether low levels of radioactivity represent DNA binding rather than spurious counts. In addition, replicate DNA extractions and assays should be performed on organ and tissue samples set aside for that purpose in order to check the reproducibility of data obtained in the first set of extractions and assays. Where there are sufficient data, a statistical analysis of DNA-binding from different tissues and organs within treatment groups may well aid in interpreting the biological significance of the results. It is not practicable to prescribe a particular method of statistical analysis without detailed knowledge of a particular set of data.

Evidence of a relationship between dose and DNA-binding is further reassurance that the radioactivity associated with DNA represents true binding. However, it is probable that experiments using several doses will not be performed and dose–response curves will not be available in the majority of cases. Where multiple doses have been used, the existence of a significant correlation can be tested by some form of regression analysis of the types discussed in *UKEMS Sub-committee on Guidelines for Mutagenicity Testing Part III* (1989). The unit of measurement to be entered into such an analysis is the specific binding, e.g. dpm/mg per organ or tissue per individual animal.

Results for levels of apparent macromolecular binding are considered in conjunction with chromatographic and other data when interpreting any possible biological significance.

4.3.3 Presentation of results

The following data should be presented:

- Details of the test compound including name, code name or code number (if used), chemical structure, chemical purity, method of synthesis; radiochemical purity, position and type of radionuclide, specific activity, method of storage, solvent, formulation of administered dose, time of formulation, time of administration.
- Species, strain, sex, age, weight, numbers and identification of animals used.
- Elapsed time between administration of test compound to killing of animals and recovery of organs.
- Types and numbers of organs and tissues recovered.
- Yield of DNA from each organ or tissue, UV spectra, estimates of purity.

Scintillation counting data: type of counter, type of scintillant and method of calibration and quench correction, amount of DNA counted per scintillation vial, raw cpm per vial, dpm per vial after correction for efficiency of counting, unit weight of bound product per unit weight of DNA, e.g. ng or μg bound per mg or g DNA, conversion to molar equivalents, e.g. moles bound per million nucleotides, summary tables showing binding data for each replicate organ in each animal at each dose point in ascending order of dose. Results for radioactivity levels associated with each organ at each time point should be the mean ± SD of at least three animals and should be expressed as % dose administered, dpm/gm of organ and dpm/organ.

Details of DNA digestion and chromatography: conditions of enzymic digestion, type of HPLC column and equipment, details of solvents, copies of HPLC profiles and digitized transformations, if available, e.g. cpm and dpm per peak; integrals of absorption, details of radioactivity measurements (see above), plots of radioactivity and UV absorption.

4.3.4 Interpretation of data in terms of positive and negative

Fig. 4.2 shows a decision tree which can be used not only for designing a DNA binding experiment but also for interpreting the results of such an experiment.

A decisively *negative* result can be claimed when none of the DNA samples contains any radioactivity above the levels obtained in animals dosed with the vehicle alone.

Where one or more samples contain counts above background, and where, after using at least two different solvent systems, it is clear that the counts co-chromatograph with normal deoxyribonucleosides, the assay can be regarded as *negative* because the counts represent metabolic incorporation rather than covalent binding.

A result is regarded as *equivocal* when *all* the counts appear in the void volume. These counts may represent incomplete digestion of adducted DNA, cross-linking of DNA to protein, or a variety of phenomena for which there is as yet no explanation. Suggestions for further studies to be performed when all the counts elute in the void volume are shown in Table 4.1.

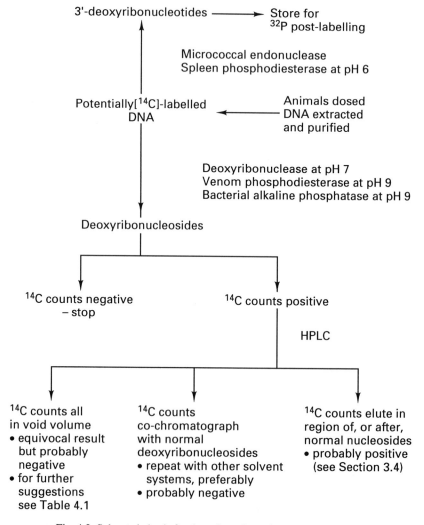

Fig. 4.2. Schematic basis for detection of covalent reaction of a [^{14}C]-labelled chemical with DNA *in vivo*.

Table 4.1. *Procedures which may be adopted if radioactivity elutes from a chromatography column with the void volume*

1. Vary the conditions and components of enzymic hydrolysis
2. Repeat chromatography using a different matrix, for example, one which allows identification of the molecular weight of radiolabelled material. It is important that any system used can adequately separate the normal DNA bases or nucleosides from the void volume
3. Perform solvent partitioning experiments
4. Perform ^{32}P labelling studies and look for migration of radioactivity on TLC
5. Hypothesise on a possible activated intermediate of the test article and synthesise this chemically. The synthesis should preferably be performed using radiolabelled compound. Attempt reaction of the intermediate with DNA and subject any product to the above studies

An experiment is *positive* when the counts elute in the region of normal deoxyribonucleosides (but do not co-chromatograph with them, see 2. in Table 4.1, above), or when the counts elute after the normal deoxyribonucleosides.

A negative control showing true radioactive contamination would invalidate the study.

Where used, a positive control must show the expected tissue distribution of radioactivity. Treatment groups should show a reasonable correlation between the dose administered and the radioactivity recovered in organs plus urine and faeces.

4.4   CONCLUSIONS AND SUMMARY

1. The detection and quantitation of DNA binding following dosing of laboratory animals with radiolabelled test compounds is a measure of the effective dose received by a particular target rather than a measure of biological effect.
2. This technique will not detect the effects of mutagens or carcinogens, or their metabolites, that do not covalently react with DNA.
3. In most cases, it should be possible to distinguish clearly between positive and negative results. However, non-specific binding of radiolabel can be a problem. The Working Group concluded that further investigation using high-performance liquid chromatography would resolve such problems in the majority of cases. It is recommended, therefore, that where radiolabelling of DNA is detected, labelled DNA is digested under appropriate conditions and subjected to HPLC analysis in order to determine the nature of the binding.

APPENDIX 4.1
EXAMPLE PROTOCOL

As an example it will be assumed that rats are the chosen species, the route of administration is by gavage and the test article is soluble in water.

Male random-bred Sprague–Dawley rats are housed in pairs in polypropylene cages with wire mesh lids and floors. Bottled mains tap water and appropriate diet are provided *ad libitum*.

Twenty-four healthy rats are used in the DNA binding assay after a period of 5 days acclimatisation. Before dosing, the selected rats are ear-tagged and allotted to four groups of six animals using a system of random numbers. Group weights are checked one day prior to treatment to ensure individual group weights differ from the mean by no more than 5%. The weight range of the animals used in the DNA binding study should normally be 150–250 g. [^{14}C]-labelled test article is used at a concentration of 1 mCi/ml with a radiochemical purity of 99.5%. The [^{14}C] test article is diluted immediately before dosing to give 200 μCi/ml (4 mg/ml). Isotonic saline is used as the diluent. Samples of the diluted solution are frozen and returned for radiochemical re-analysis.

Dosing of animals

Animals are weighed before dosing and the volume of vehicle or [^{14}C] test article solution to be administered is calculated based on a dose volume of say 10 ml/kg. The actual dose of [^{14}C]-labelled test article administered is 40 mg/kg, or 2 mCi/kg.

The test article is administered, using a stainless steel gavage needle, orally as a single dose to each of 18 rats. DNA binding is determined after 6, 24 and 48 hours exposure (times based on knowledge of the metabolism of the test article). One group of six animals is administered vehicle control and serves as the negative control to be sacrificed after 48 h.

Collection of urine and faeces

The 48-hour group is placed in wire-floored, glass metabolism cages the day before dosing. Urine and faeces collected within the apparatus are removed at four time points: immediately before dosing, and at 6, 24 and 48 hours afterwards. Collection vessels are replaced with clean ones at the 6 hour time-point. The volumes of the urines and weights of faeces are determined, and small samples of each taken for radioactivity determination. The bulk of the urine and faeces are stored frozen at −90 °C.

Rats are removed from the metabolism cages 48 hours after treatment. The interior of each cage is then flushed through with approximately 500 ml of methanol. These washings are stored at 4 °C before concentration by flash evaporation and determination of radioactivity.

Killing of animals and collection of tissues

Rats treated with [^{14}C]-labelled test article, are killed in groups of six after 6, 24 and 48 hours; vehicle-treated rats are killed after 48 hours. Animals are killed by asphyxiation with carbon dioxide, following the order in which they were dosed.

Animals are pinned to dissection boards protected from contamination by fresh paper towelling. To check for any contamination of the autopsy area that might have occurred during processing of the treated animals, various surfaces are swabbed with methanol-soaked filter disks between killing of different groups. The radioactivity of the disks is determined. Dissecting instruments are cleaned with RBS or similar detergent between killing of each group to prevent cross-contamination with radioactive material. A fresh set of instruments is used for the excision of organs from untreated animals which are dissected last (lack of radioactivity in these samples provides evidence that no cross-contamination has occurred).

Stomach, small intestine, kidneys, liver and colon are removed. Stomachs are opened by longitudinal section of the greater curve and the contents removed by flushing with ice cold 150 mM KCl. Lengths of small intestine and colon are cleared by mechanical extrusion, followed by flushing with cold 150 mM KCl via a syringe. The organs are then placed in tubes containing 15 ml ice-cold 150 mM KCl. All organs are then washed twice with approximately 50 ml of ice-cold 150 mM KCl and blotted to remove excess liquid. Organs are weighed, wrapped in labelled foil, rapidly frozen in liquid nitrogen, placed in secondary containers marked with study number and kill time, and stored at -90 °C until required for analysis.

Bone marrow is obtained by exposing both femurs, removing them and cleaning adherent tissue. The shank is cut from the ends using bone clippers. Appropriately labelled disposable centrifuge tubes are filled with 2 ml each of ice-cold 150 mM KCl. Some of this solution is drawn into a 1 ml syringe with a fresh needle and used to aspirate the contents of each femur into the appropriate centrifuge tube.

The tubes are centrifuged at 200 G for 5 minutes at 4 °C. Supernatants are decanted, the pellets are resuspended in 10 ml of 150 mM KCl and centrifuged again. This process is repeated and pellets are stored at -90 °C until required for analysis.

Determination of radioactivity in urine, faeces and cage washes
Urine

Samples of urine are diluted 1000-fold with distilled water. Aliquots of this dilution (1.0 ml) are added to 4.0 ml scintillant. Vials are counted using a scintillation counter with automatic quench correction by external standardisation. The large dilution of the urine sample obviates the need for decolourising the material.

Faeces

A weighed sample (100 mg) is hand homogenised in 1 ml distilled water. Aliquots (0.1 ml) of each suspension are added to 0.9 ml scintillant compatible tissue solubiliser and allowed to incubate until solution is achieved. Of this solution, 0.1 ml is added to 4.5 ml scintillant for counting. Quench correction is by external standardisation using a stored quench curve.

Cage washes

The evaporated residues of the methanol washes from the metabolism cages are redissolved in 20 ml of methanol. A 0.1 ml sample of these solutions is diluted with 0.4 ml of 150 mM KCl, and added to scintillant for determination of radioactivity.

Processing of whole organs prior to extraction of macromolecules

It is useful to determine the tissue distribution of the test article. Organs are thawed and small samples of known weight (approximately 100 mg is adequate) removed and solubilised for determination of radioactivity. Each sample is added to 1 ml of tissue solubiliser and left to dissolve. Scintillation counting and quench correction are as described for faecal samples. It is equally acceptable to process these samples as tissue homogenates. In this case, the tissue sample is hand homogenised with 1 ml of 150 mM KCl. A sample (0.5 ml) of this suspension, further diluted 1:4 (v/v) with 150 mM KCl if necessary, is added to scintillant. To correct for quenching, an internal standard, usually at least 10^4 dpm of [^{14}C]-toluene, is added. The ratio of the increase in sample cpm to the dpm of standard added is the efficiency of counting in the sample. This value is used to correct the sample cpm value to dpm.

Extraction and purification of DNA

DNA is extracted from liver, small intestine, colon and kidneys (both kidneys from each animal) from at least three animals of each group. Unused organs from the remaining animals are kept in store at -90 °C. For small organs pooling from more animals may be required. Extraction of DNA can be performed on the whole organ or on isolated nuclei (Croy *et al.*, 1978). In the present example, DNA extraction from intact organ tissue is described.

Hydroxylapatite method

This procedure is preferred as the one capable of providing the purest DNA. However, there is great variation in the efficacy of different preparations of hydroxylapatite for this application and all batches should be validated using commercially produced DNA before use in an assay. The procedure is described below using liver as an example organ, e.g. Beland, Dooley & Casiano, (1979) and Martin *et al.*, (1982).

Each liver is transferred to a large centrifuge tube to which 20 ml of phosphate buffered urea : sodium dodecyl sulphate : ethylenediamine tetraacetic acid (MUPSE; see Appendix 4.2) is added. Whilst being kept on ice, the tissue is chopped with scissors and then homogenised using an Ultraturrax (or similar) blender at full speed. It is desirable to use 20-second bursts with a period between to allow recooling. The suspension is poured out and a further 30 ml of MUPSE used to wash the homogeniser probe. This wash is added to the original homogenate. An equal volume of MUPSE-saturated chloroform : isoamyl alcohol : phenol (CIP, see Appendix 4.2) is added. The mixture is stirred at room temperature for 3 minutes, divided between two centrifuge tubes and then centrifuged at approximately 2000 G for 10 minutes at 20 °C. The lower layer is removed, using a submerged pipette, and discarded. The upper white layer is extracted twice more by making up to 50 ml with MUPSE-saturated CIP and mixed for 1 minute before centrifuging again. An equal volume of diethyl ether is then added to each tube and the two layers thoroughly mixed by repeated inversion. Samples are centrifuged at approximately 2000 G for 10 minutes and the upper organic layer discarded. The ether extraction is repeated and the lower aqueous layers pooled from the two centrifuge tubes. The sample is then applied to an hydroxylapatite column prepared as described in Appendix 4.3. The sample is applied at a flow rate of 2 ml per minute. The column is then washed with MUP (see Appendices 4.1 and 4.3) at 2 ml per minute until the monitored absorbance of the eluate at 254 nm returns to the baseline. The column is washed with 0.014 M sodium phosphate (pH 6.8) at 2 ml/min for 30 minutes, then DNA is eluted with 0.48 M sodium phosphate (pH 6.8) at 2 ml/min.

The DNA-containing eluate is dialysed using Visking tubing against 2×5 litres of distilled water for a total of at least 16 hours. Each dialysate is reduced in volume by rotary evaporation to approximately 15 ml. This solution is dialysed against 250 ml of 5 mM Bis Tris pH 7.1 for at least two hours. To the solution is added 1/10 volume of 1 M NaCl. It is then made up to 50 ml with ice-cold ethanol.

The precipitated DNA is either removed immediately or after storage overnight at -20 °C. The DNA is collected by centrifugation at approximately 1200 G for 10 minutes. The pellet is dissolved in 2 ml 50 mM Bis Tris pH 7.1 containing 5 mM $MgCl_2$ and stored at -20 °C until required for analysis. DNA prepared by this method has been shown to be highly pure with less than 0.1% contamination by RNA or protein.

Enzymic method

The recovery of RNA and protein are not within the scope of this chapter, however, the choice of DNA extraction method may be influenced, in part, by the desire to evaluate binding to protein or RNA. For recovery of RNA, the enzymic method is perhaps favourable.

The following description of an enzymic methodology applies to 10 g of tissue. Volumes are adjusted according to the actual weight of the organ, e.g. see Benson, Martin & Garner, (1988).

Organ samples are added to a centrifuge tube and 50 ml of 1 mM EDTA/ 10% SDS added per 10 g tissue. The tissue is homogenised using an Ultraturrax blender. The homogenate is centrifuged sufficiently (at least 700 G for 10 minutes) to disperse any foam. Proteinase K is added (1.25 ml of 10 mg/ml solution per tube) and the mixture incubated at 37 °C for 30 minutes. Each tube is made up to 50 ml with phenol reagent (phenol crystals saturated with 50 mM Tris HCl, pH 8.0) and mixed for a few minutes. The mixture is separated into layers by centrifuging at 1250–2000 G for 10 minutes. It is recommended that the phenol layer be retained if extraction of protein is to be performed. Further extractions of the aqueous layer are made with 50 ml phenol : chloroform : isoamyl alcohol (25 : 24 : 1, v/v), followed by Tris saturated chloroform : isoamyl alcohol (24 : 1, v/v). In each case, the two layers are separated by centrifugation at approximately 2000 G for 5–10 minutes. To the aqueous layer is added 5 M NaCl (5 ml) and DNA is precipitated by the addition of 120–150 ml ice-cold ethanol or 2-ethoxyethanol, the latter being used where an RNA fraction is required. The DNA is washed twice with 70% ethanol and then dissolved in 10 ml of SSC–EDTA buffer (1.5 mM NaCl : 0.15 mM trisodium citrate : 1 mM EDTA) for RNAase treatment. To this solution is added 0.1 ml of 1 M Tris HCl pH 7.4, 750 units of RNAase T1 (this is an excess and is irrespective of organ type and weight except for very small organ samples) and 1.5 ml of heat-treated RNAase A (1 mg/ml). The mixture is incubated for 15 minutes at 37 °C. Further 1 M Tris-HCl (pH 8.0, 0.625 ml) is added and enzymic proteins extracted from the mixture using 15 ml portions of phenol : chloroform : isoamyl alcohol

(25 : 24 : 1, v/v) followed by chloroform : isoamyl alcohol (24 : 1, v/v) as described above. DNA is recovered by addition of 1.5 ml of 1 M NaCl followed by ice-cold ethanol to 50 ml. Where necessary, complete precipitation is aided by placing at -90 °C overnight. The pellet is harvested by centrifugation at 1000–2000 G for 10 minutes and washed sequentially with ethanol, ethanol : acetone (1 : 1, v/v) and acetone leaving the pellet to soak in each for at least 15 minutes. After each wash, DNA is recovered by appropriate centrifugation, e.g. 700–1225 G for 5–10 minutes). The DNA is dried using a stream of nitrogen and, if not quantified immediately, is stored at -20 °C until required.

Quantification of DNA

Irrespective of organ of origin, extracted DNA samples are dissolved in a suitable volume (2–4 ml) of 50 mM Bis Tris/5 mM MgCl$_2$, pH 7.1. If necessary (for example if the animal was not starved prior to and during exposure and the organ of interest is the liver) the DNA solution is ultra-centrifuged at 110 000–125 000 G for 60 minutes to remove glycogen. DNA is recovered from the supernatant by ethanol precipitation as described earlier and the DNA redissolved in 50 mM Bis Tris/5 mM MgCl$_2$, pH 7.1. Samples of DNA solutions are taken for scintillation counting as described below. Further samples (25–100 µl, depending on the DNA content expected) are taken and made up to 1 ml in 5% w/v trichloracetic acid. DNA is hydrolysed by heating at 90 °C for 20 minutes. After cooling, 2 ml of Burton diphenylamine reagent (Appendix 4.4) is added and colour developed overnight in the dark. The absorbance of the sample at 600 nm is determined and DNA content is calculated using a standard curve prepared simultaneously with known concentrations of hydrolysed calf thymus DNA (Appendix 4.4).

Determination of DNA radioactivity

Solutions of extracted DNA are prepared for scintillation counting by DNAase I digestion. DNAase is added to at least three samples of each DNA solution, typically 0.1, 0.2, and 0.4 ml, but also 0.8 ml if the DNA concentration is low. DNAase is added at the rate of at least 0.1 µg/mg DNA and samples are incubated at 37 °C for 15–30 minutes. Scintillant is then added and samples counted for [^{14}C] activity.

From the concentration of DNA in the sample and its radioactivity, values for apparent DNA binding are calculated.

Hydrolysis of DNA

If radiolabel is found associated with the DNA then the nature of such association needs to be established.

There are four possibilities:

Table 4.2

Step	Enzyme	Addition/mg DNA	Incubation period at 37 °C
1	DNAase	200 units	At least 3 hours
2	Nuclease P_1	20 μl of 0.5 mg/ml solution in 1 mM $MgCl_2$	From 3 hours after addition of DNAase I, continuing overnight
	Alkaline phosphatase	2 unit	
	Acid phosphatase	0.5 units	
	Snake venom phosphodiesterase	0.001–0.005 units	

1. The test article is covalently bound to DNA producing an adduct with one or more of the four bases at one or more positions of substitution.
2. The radioactivity is associated non-covalently with DNA; this is unlikely if the above extraction techniques have been used, and especially so if the hydroxylapatite method has been used.
3. The radioactivity has been incorporated into one or more of the DNA nucleotides by a combination of metabolism and catabolism.
4. The radioactivity is associated with a persistent contaminant of the DNA sample, for example, tightly bound protein which has survived the purification procedure.

Possibility 4. can be addressed by determination of the extent of protein contamination and the extent of binding to protein. It is more difficult to discriminate between possibilities 1. and 3.

It is beyond the scope of this chapter to discuss details of methodology of the many research techniques which can be applied to address this problem but a brief mention of the techniques follows.

If a putative pathway of metabolism can be defined, the proposed activated metabolites should be synthesised and reacted under appropriate conditions with naked DNA. Any adducts obtained following appropriate hydrolysis of the DNA should be purified and used as chromatography markers. The DNA from the study is then similarly hydrolysed and co-injected onto a suitable chromatography system. The relationship of eluted radioactivity and UV absorbing material at an appropriate wavelength is then monitored. Similar behaviour of the synthetic adduct(s) and radiolabelled material from hydrolysed sample DNA is then sought in other systems, e.g. solvent partitioning (Beland *et al.*, 1979).

If, after appropriate hydrolysis, the radioactivity associated with the DNA from the study co-chromatographs in at least two systems with one or more of the normal DNA components then it may be assumed that possibility 3., namely metabolic incorporation, is likely.

Where enzymic hydrolysis is to be used, DNA solutions are diluted, where possible, to 2 mg/ml with 50 mM Bis Tris/5 mM $MgCl_2$, pH 7.1 and hydrolysed as detailed in Table 4.2.

The activity of the enzymes used is confirmed by a control hydrolysis of calf thymus DNA concurrently with the experimental samples. Hydrolysates are stored at 4 °C to await chromatographic analysis.

Where acid hydrolysis is to be used, the DNA must be dissolved in a very weak buffer which is then made 0.1 M with respect to HCl. The precipitate is then heated at 70 °C for 20 minutes to depurinate the DNA.

APPENDIX 4.2
DNA PURIFICATION REAGENTS
(HYDROXYLAPATITE METHOD)

MUP–SDS–EDTA (MUPSE)

Chemical	Wt/litre	Final conc.	
Urea	480.5 g	8.0	M
$NaH_2PO_4.2H_2O$	37.4 g	0.24	M
SDS	10.0 g	0.035	M
Disodium EDTA.$2H_2O$	3.7 g	0.01	M
Distilled water	500 ml in first instance		

pH is adjusted to 6.8 with concentrated NaOH and then made up to 1 litre with distilled water.

MUP

Urea	480.5 g	8.0	M
$NaH_2PO_4.2H_2O$	37.4 g	0.24	M
Distilled water	500 ml in first instance		

pH is adjusted to 6.8 with concentrated NaOH and then made up to 1 litre with distilled water.

Chloroform–isoamyl alcohol–phenol (CIP)

Chloroform	480.0 ml
Isoamyl alcohol	20.0 ml
Phenol (crystals)	500.0 g

APPENDIX 4.3
PREPARATION OF HYDROXYLAPATITE
COLUMNS

Columns are prepared using at least 1 g of DNA grade hydroxy-lapatite per 1 g net weight of the organ to be processed. In this example, organs are assumed to be 10 g. For other weights amounts are adjusted pro rata.

Approximately 15 g hydroxylapatite are suspended in 100 ml of 0.014 M sodium phosphate buffer, pH 6.8. The suspension is heated at 85 °C for 15 minutes. After cooling and swirling, the slurry is left to settle for a few minutes. The fines are decanted off and the process repeated with 100 ml MUP. The MUP slurry is poured into a 2.6 × 40 cm glass chromatography column and 100 ml MUP is pumped through at a flow rate of 2–4 ml per minute until the UV absorbance at 254 nm of the eluent is constant.

APPENDIX 4.4
REAGENTS FOR QUANTITATION OF DNA
Standards for colourimetric DNA determination

A stock solution of calf thymus DNA is accurately prepared at 1 mg per ml in 5% w/v TCA and heated at 90 °C for 2 minutes. This is stored at 4–8 °C until required. On the day of the determination 1.0 ml is removed and diluted with 9.0 ml of 5% w/v TCA to give a working solution of 100 μg per ml. From this a series of standards is prepared by dilution in 5% w/v TCA to a final volume of 1.0 ml. A range of standards, including a zero control, are prepared on each occasion.

Burton diphenylamine colourimetric reagent

This solution is prepared just prior to the determination by dissolving 2 g of diphenylamine in approximately 80 ml glacial acetic acid. To this, 4.4 ml of 60% v/v perchloric acid and 0.5 ml 2% v/v acetaldehyde are added. The solution is then made up to a final volume of 100 ml by further addition of glacial acetic acid.

APPENDIX 4.5
OTHER METHODS TO DETECT DNA BINDING

[32P]-post-labelling is a sensitive and non-specific technique for the detection of a wide variety of carcinogen adduct structures (Phillips, 1990*a*). It generally involves the following steps:

1. enzymic digestion of DNA to nucleoside 3'-monophosphates
2. T4 polynucleotide kinase-catalysed transfer of [32P]-orthophosphate from [gamma-32P]ATP to the 5'-position of the nucleotides

3. chromatographic separation of the [^{32}P]-labelled adducts from the normal nucleotides and resolution by thin-layer or high-performance liquid chromatography

4. detection and quantitation of the adducts by monitoring decay of ^{32}P. Standard procedures can generally achieve a detection limit of 1 adduct in 10^7 nucleotides using a few micrograms of DNA, and in certain circumstances one of a number of variations may be applicable whereby the post-labelling is specifically targeted at the adducts only, and the detection limit may be lowered to 1 adduct in 10^9–10^{10} nucleotides (Gupta, 1985; Reddy & Randerath, 1986).

At present, there are many practical difficulties which compromise its routine use. First, the technique is relatively new and has not yet achieved a sufficient degree of standardisation between laboratories that would allow the establishment of a recommended protocol. Secondly, although it is not in theory necessary to know the way in which a compound is activated and interacts with DNA in order to detect its adduct or adducts by [^{32}P]-post-labelling, in practice the dependence of the method on chromatographic separation of labelled, modified nucleotides from unmodified ones requires some predictions to be made about the likely mobility and/or hydrophobicity of a putative adduct. Not only are the chromatographic systems used to separate adducts formed by large aromatic carcinogens different from those formed by small alkylating agents (Reddy *et al.*, 1984), but some of the enhancement procedures that push the sensitivity of the labelling technique to the limits quoted are selective for certain types of adducts. Thus, for example, nuclease P1 digestion will enhance the sensitivity with which adducts formed by PAHs, but not aromatic amines and alkylating agents, can be detected, while butanol extraction improves the sensitivity of detection of adducts of PAHs and of some, but not all, aromatic amines (Gupta & Earley, 1988; Gallagher *et al.*, 1989; Hall *et al.*, 1990).

While, in principle, this method does not have an absolute requirement for synthetic standards, in practice either these or a structurally related analogue that can serve as an adduct-forming, positive control are highly desirable to avoid the possibility of a false negative (Phillips, 1990*b*). While reasonable confidence can be placed on a positive result, there is always a suspicion with a negative [^{32}P]-post-labelling result that either the chromatographic procedures or that the DNA digestion procedures were inappropriate. In addition, there is evidence that some types of adducts are not efficiently labelled with ^{32}P by T4 polynucleotide kinase (Hemminki, Peltonen & Mustonen, 1990).

Immunochemical methods of DNA adduct detection require a somewhat different approach in that it is generally necessary first to generate a sample of

DNA highly modified by a chemical moiety, then to raise monoclonal or polyclonal antibodies to it, and then to use these antibodies to detect the presence of adducts in the samples of DNA under investigation (Poirier 1981; Strickland & Boyle, 1984). The sensitivity of these methods can achieve the detection of as little as 1 adduct in 10^7–10^8 nucleotides. This approach is clearly not applicable to investigating the putative formation of DNA adducts of unknown structure by a novel chemical.

With antibodies raised against adducts of more complex structure, there is evidently an unavoidable cross-reactivity with adducts formed by carcinogenic compounds of similar structure (Phillips, 1990*a*). Thus it is possible to use a particular antibody to detect the presence of a limited range of adduct structures, an approach which could be used to test the adduct forming ability of a new compound if it were structurally related to a carcinogen, to whose DNA adducts antibodies had been produced. It will be clear from the foregoing that the methods described in this section are research techniques that are not yet ready for routine application as test procedures. Nevertheless, there may be particular combinations of circumstances that would warrant their application such as the study of putative DNA adduct formation during chronic, long-term dosing of animals.

4.5   REFERENCES

Andersson, H. C. & Kihlman, B. A. (1989). The production of chromosomal alterations in human lymphocytes by drugs known to interfere with the activity of DNA topisomerase II. I. *m*-AMSA. *Carcinogenesis*, **10**, 123–30.

Baird, W. M. & Brookes, P. (1973). Isolation of hydrocarbon-deoxyriboside products from DNA of mouse embryo cells treated in culture with 7-methylbenz(*a*)anthracene -³H. *Cancer Research*, **33**, 2378–85.

Basler, A. (1986). Aneuploidy-inducing chemicals in yeast evaluated by the micronucleus test. *Mutation Research*, **174**, 11–13.

Beland, F. A., Dooley, K. L. & Casiano, D. A. (1979). Rapid isolation of carcinogen-bound DNA and RNA by hydroxyapatite chromatography. *Journal of Chromatography*, **174**, 177–86.

Benson, A. J., Martin, C. N. & Garner, R. C. (1988). N-(2-hydroxyethyl)-N-[2-(7-guaninyl)ethyl]amine, the putative major DNA adduct of cyclophosphamide *in vitro* and *in vivo* in the rat. *Biochemical Pharmacology*, **37**, 2979–85.

Cooper, C. S. & Grover, P. L. (eds.) (1990). *Chemical Carcinogenesis and Mutagenesis I. Handbook of Experimental Pharmacology*, volume 94/1, Springer-Verlag, Berlin.

Croy, R. G., Essigman, J. M., Reinhold, V. N. & Wogan, G. N. (1978). Identification of the principal aflatoxin B_1-DNA adduct formed *in vivo* in rat liver. *Proceedings of the National Academy of Sciences, USA*, **75**, 1745–9.

Degraeve, N. (1978). Genetic and related effects of Vinca rosea alkaloids. *Mutation Research*, **55**, 31–42.

DeMarini, D. M., Brock, K. H., Doerr, C. L. & Moore, M. M. (1987). Mutagenicity and clastogenicity of teniposide (VM-26) in L5178Y TK+/− -3.7.2C mouse lymphoma cells. *Mutation Research*, **187**, 141–9.

Dring, L. G. (1987). Methods for studying metabolism and distribution *in vivo* of radiolabelled drugs. In *Biochemical Toxicology – A Practical Approach*, eds. K. Snell and B. Mullock, IRL Press, Oxford, pp. 3–21.

Ehling, U. H., Kratochvilova, J., Lehmacher, W. & Neuhauser-Klaus, A. (1988). Mutagenicity testing of vincristine sulfate in germ cells of male mice. *Mutation Research*, **209**, 107–13.

Gallagher, J. E., Jackson, M. A., George, M. H., Lewtas, J., Robertson, I. G. C. (1989). Differences in detection of DNA adducts in the [^{32}P]-postlabelling assay after either 1-butanol extraction or nuclease P1 treatment. *Cancer Letters*, **45**, 7–12.

Grover, P. L., ed. (1979). *Chemical Carcinogenesis and DNA*, vols. I and II, CRC Press Inc., Boca Raton, Florida, USA.

Gupta, R. C. (1985). Enhanced sensitivity of [^{32}P]-postlabeling analysis of aromatic carcinogen : DNA adducts. *Cancer Research*, **45**, 5656–62.

Gupta, R. S., Bromke, A., Bryant, D. W., Gupta, R., Singh, B. & McCalla, D. R. (1987). Etoposide (VP16) and teniposide (VM26): novel anticancer drugs, strongly mutagenic in mammalian but not in prokaryotic test systems. *Mutagenesis*, **2**, 179–86.

Gupta, R. C. & Earley, K. (1988). [^{32}P]-adduct assay: comparative recoveries of structurally diverse DNA adducts in the various enhancement procedures. *Carcinogenesis*, **9**, 1687–93.

Hall, M., Ni She, M., Wild, D., Fasshauer, I., Hewer A. & Phillips, D. H. (1990). Tissue distribution of DNA adducts in CDF1 mice fed 2-amino-3-methylimidazo[4,5-f]quinoline (IQ) and 2-amino-3,4-dimethylimidazo[4,5-f]quinoline (MeIQ). *Carcinogenesis*, **11**, 1005–11.

Hemminki, K., Peltonen, K. & Mustonen, R. (1990). [^{32}P]-postlabelling of 7-methyl-dGMP and platinated dGpdG. *Chemical–Biological Interactions*, **74**, 45–54.

Kunz, B. A. (1988). Mutagenesis and deoxyribonucleotide pool imbalance. *Mutation Research*, **200**, 133–47.

Martin, C. N., Beland, F. A., Roth, R. W. & Kadlubar, F. F. (1982). Covalent binding of benzidine and N-acetylbenzidine to DNA at the C-8 atom of deoxyguanosine *in vivo* and *in vitro*. *Cancer Research*, **42**, 2678–86.

Martin, C. N. & Jennings, G. S. (1990). Comparison of the mutagenic potency of DNA adducts formed by reactive derivatives of aflatoxin, benzidine and 1-nitropyrene in a plasmid system. In *Nitroarenes*, ed. P. C. Howard, Plenum Press, New York, USA, pp. 157–66.

Muraoka, Y., Takita, T. & Umezawa, H. (1986). Bleomycin and peplomycin. In *Cancer Chemotherapy*, vol. 8, eds. H. M. Pinedo and B. A. Chabner, Elsevier, Amsterdam, pp. 65–72.

Onfelt, A. (1986). Mechanistic aspects of chemical induction of spindle disturbances and abnormal chromosome numbers. *Mutation Research*, **168**, 249–300.

Osborne, M. R. & Crosby, N. T. (1987). *Benzopyrenes*, Cambridge University Press, Cambridge, pp. 148–52.

Osborne, M. R. (1984). In *Chemical Carcinogens*, 2nd edn, vol. I, ed. C. E. Searle, American Chemical Society, Washington, pp. 485–575.

Phillips, D. H. (1990*a*). Further evidence that eugenol does not bind to DNA *in vivo*. *Mutation Research*, **245**, 23–6.

Phillips, D. H. (1990*b*). Modern methods of DNA adduct determination. In *Chemical Carcinogenesis and Mutagenesis I, Handbook of Experimental Pharmacology*, vol. 94/I, eds. C. S. Cooper and P. L. Grover, Berlin, Springer-Verlag, pp. 503–46.

Poirier, M. C. (1981). Antibodies to carcinogen–DNA adducts. *Journal of the National Cancer Institute*, **67**, 515–19.

Reddy, M. V., Gupta, R. C., Randerath, E. & Randerath, K. (1984). [^{32}P]-postlabelling test for covalent DNA binding of chemicals *in vivo*: application to a variety of aromatic carcinogens and methylating agents. *Carcinogenesis*, **5**, 231–43.

Reddy, M. V. & Randerath, K. (1986). Nuclease P1-mediated enhancement of sensitivity of [^{32}P]-postlabelling test for structurally diverse DNA adducts. *Carcinogenesis*, **7**, 1543–51.

Rohrborn, G. & Basler, A. (1981). *In vitro* and *in vivo* studies on possible mutagenic effects of the Vinca alkloid vindesine sulfate. In *Proceedings of the International Vinca Alkaloid Symposium – Vindesine*, eds. W. Brade, G. A. Nagel and S. Seeber, S. Marger, Basel, pp. 43–52.

Ross, W. E., Sullivan, D. M. & Chow, K.-C. (1988). Altered function of DNA topoisomerases as a basis for antineoplastic drug action. In *Important Advances in Oncology*, eds. V. T. De Vita, S. Hellman and S. A. Rosenberg, J. P. Lippincot, Philadelphia, pp. 65–81.

Searle, C. W., ed. (1984). *Chemical Carcinogens*, 2nd edn, vols. I and II, American Chemical Society, Washington.

Shooter, K. V. (1978). DNA phosphotriesters as indicators of cumulative carcinogen-induced damage. *Nature*, **274**, 612–14.

Sowers, L. C., Eritja, R., Kaplan, B., Goodman, M. F. & Fazakerly, G. V. (1988). Equilibrium between a wobble and ionized base pair formed between fluorouracil and guanine in DNA as studied by proton and fluorine NMR. *Journal of Biological Chemistry*, **263**, 14794–801.

Strickland, P. T. & Boyle, J. M. (1984). Immunoassay of carcinogen modified DNA. *Progress in Nucleic Acid Research Molecular Biology*, **31**, 1–58.

Swenson, D. H. & Lawley, P. D. (1978). Alkylation of DNA by carcinogens dimethyl sulphate, ethyl methanesulphonate, *N*-ethyl-*N*-nitrosourea and *N*-methyl-*N*-nitrosourea: relative reactivity of the phosphodiester site thymidylyl (3'-5') thymidine. *Biochemical Journal*, **171**, 575–87.

UKEMS Sub-committee on Guidelines for Mutagenicity Testing, Report. (1989). Part III *Statistical Evaluation of Mutagenicity Test Data*, ed. D. J. Kirkland, Cambridge University Press, Cambridge.

UKEMS Sub-committee on Guidelines for Mutagenicity Testing, Report. (1990) Part I *Revised Basic Mutagenicity Tests*, ed. D. J. Kirkland, Cambridge University Press, Cambridge.

5

Mammalian germ cell cytogenetics

C. Tease   E. P. Evans   J. M. Mackay

5.1   INTRODUCTION

Germ cell cytogenetic tests are neither a necessary nor desirable part of the initial screening programme for potential genotoxins. Rather, they are usually undertaken as supplementary investigations of compounds that have been previously assessed for genotoxicity in *in vitro* tests and somatic cell assays *in vivo*. To date, no compound has been found whose mutagenic effect is limited to germ cells (Holden, 1982). Thus all compounds that have proved positive in a germ cell test also gave a positive response in *in vitro* tests and somatic cell assays *in vivo*. Currently, therefore, there is no reason to suspect that these latter assays will not also identify compounds with the potential to cause heritable genetic damage. It is important to realise, however, that not all compounds that prove mutagenic in somatic cell assays behave similarly in germ cell tests. Indeed, only a relatively small number of chemicals are known to induce gene mutations in the germ line (Russell & Shelby, 1985) although this is undoubtedly related to the comparatively small proportion of compounds that have been examined in such tests. Moreover, the degree of genetic damage observed in *in vitro* tests and somatic cell assays *in vivo* has not been found to correlate consistently with that in a germ cell test. Thus at present, there is no reliable means of predicting from *in vitro* tests and somatic cell assays *in vivo* the likely response of germ cells to any particular compound. This problem is in large part due to the complex biology of germ cells and to the sex-related differences in germ cell development.

Overall, it is recommended that germ cell tests should only be undertaken where it is important to obtain direct information on the response of germ cells to a substance that has been shown by *in vitro* and somatic cell assays to be mutagenic and also been shown by radiolabelled pharmacokinetic studies to penetrate the germinal tissue. The cytogenetic tests described here provide a comparatively rapid and efficient approach to investigation of germ cell effects.

5.1.1   Principles and genetic basis

The cytogenetic tests are designed to detect and quantify numerical and structural chromosome aberrations occurring either spontaneously or induced in germ line cells by genotoxic compounds. These anomalies can be assayed directly in the cells in which they arose, at subsequent stages of germ cell development, or in the resulting embryos and liveborn progeny.

5.1.2   Germ cell development

In order to undertake germ cell tests it is essential to have at the very least a basic knowledge of the organisation of the testis and ovary and also of the process of meiosis which is central to the production of gametes. The brief descriptions below provide an introduction to mammalian germ cell biology which should be useful for a fuller appreciation of the strengths and limitations of the various tests. Throughout the report, the mouse is used as the model species as it is the most commonly used and many of the tests were initially developed for this species. Where possible, however, references for other species are given to provide access to the relevant literature.

5.1.2.1   *Spermatogenesis*

Primordial germ cells can be recognised during very early embryonic stages of both sexes (day 8 of gestation in the mouse) by their characteristic appearance and staining properties (Setchell, 1978). These primordial germ cells migrate from the dorsal endoderm of the yolk sac to the urogenital ridge where they are incorporated into the developing gonad and a short time later (by day 12 of gestation) sexual differentiation is clearly visible (for review see Byskov, 1982). The embryonic cells that give rise to the male germ cells are called spermatogonia. These immature germ cells have a diploid genome and divide mitotically. Spermatogonial mitosis effectively ceases during late foetal life and is only re-initiated after birth (Oakberg, 1981).

The testis contains self-renewing, stem cell populations of spermatogonia (A_s cells) located in the basal compartment of the testicular tubules; A_s cells, by mitotic division, give rise to three types of differentiating spermatogonia: A, Intermediate and B (Setchell, 1978). A cells are generally believed to have a relatively long cell cycle and therefore represent only a small fraction of the mitoses seen in a testicular preparation, the majority being the more actively dividing differentiating spermatogonial stages (Oakberg, 1956; Monesi, 1962; Adler & Brewen, 1982).

Immediately after the final mitotic division of the differentiating B spermatogonia, the cells commence meiosis at which stage they are called spermatocytes. Cells in the first meiotic division are termed primary spermatocytes and those in the second meiotic division are called secondary spermatocytes (Setchell, 1978). The meiotic maturation stages between primary and secondary spermatocytes are well defined. In the mouse it takes approximately 12–14 days for primary spermatocytes to mature from the pre-meiotic S phase to the diakinesis/metaphase I stage of meiosis with the second meiotic division following several hours later (Oakberg, 1960). Following the completion of the second meiotic division spermatids are formed and these then undergo complex biochemical and morphological changes to differentiate into mature spermatozoa (Setchell, 1978). The whole process from spermato-gonial stem cell to mature spermatozoon takes approximately 42 days in the mouse (Oakberg, 1956).

5.1.2.2 Oogenesis

In contrast to events in the testis, female germ cells enter meiosis during gestation (or shortly after birth in the cases of a few mammals such as the rabbit) after a limited number of mitotic divisions (Peters & McNatty, 1980). Most importantly, unlike the male, there is no self-renewing stem cell component and so the ovary contains the life-time supply of oocytes at birth. Oocytes enter meiosis from approximately day 13 of gestation and over a period of a few days all the germ cells become committed to meiosis (Speed, 1982; Dietrich, 1986). The cells progress through the early stages of prophase I until they reach diplotene at which stage they enter a developmental arrest. The chromosomes take on a very diffuse appearance and cells in this condition are termed dictyate. At birth or very shortly thereafter all the germ cells have achieved the dictyate state. The chromosomes retain this diffuse appearance until a few hours prior to ovulation when meiosis is re-initiated in response to a gonadotrophic hormone signal.

The ovary of a sexually mature female consists of a pool of primary, immature oocytes from which cells are selected at regular intervals for growth and maturation. The process by which cells are selected is not understood. Immature oocytes are surrounded by a layer of somatic cells. After selection of the germ cell for maturation the associated somatic cells increase in numbers and form a complex organelle, the follicle, which plays an important role in steroidogenesis. The exact time required for an oocyte to transit from initial selection through to ovulation has proved difficult to determine in any mammalian species for technical reasons. The best data on this come from the mouse in which the process is believed to take more than 7 weeks (Oakberg, 1979).

Following the cyclical surge of gonadotrophic hormones, oocytes in mature (Graafian) follicles re-enter the meiotic division. The cells rapidly complete the first meiotic division but arrest once more at metaphase II. Release from this second phase of arrest comes when the egg is fertilised and this stimulus allows the cell to complete meiosis.

5.1.2.3 *Embryogenesis*

Successful fertilisation of an ovum by a spermatozoon results in the union of the male and female pronuclei to restore the diploid chromosome number for the beginning of embryogenesis. Although small differences in the timing of embryonic stages may occur between inbred mouse strains or in hybrids between them, nevertheless a generalised description of embryo-genesis can be made (Rugh, 1968; Hogan, Constantini & Lacy, 1986; Thieler, 1989).

Mice normally mate during the middle of the dark period of the diurnal cycle and the mating is marked by the coagulation of the male ejaculate in the vagina of the female to form a copulation plug. The most frequently used convention describes the day on which the copulation plug is found as day 0 of pregnancy and the embryos as being half-day post-coitum (p.c.) in development. The one-cell embryo undergoes its first cleavage division during day 1 p.c. to form a two-cell (two blastomere) egg. Further divisions give rise to a 4 to 16 cell morula by day 2 p.c. During the course of day 3, the morula develops into the blastocyst which when fully expanded contains about 64 cells. The blastocyst sheds its zona pellucida and implants in the uterus at about day 4.5 p.c.; this event marks the end of the pre-implantation stage and the beginning of the post-implantation stage of development. It should be noted that embryos are not fully synchronised in their development, moreover, chromosomally abnormal embryos, such as monosomics, may show significant developmental retardation even at these early stages (Beechey & Searle, 1988).

Shortly after implantation, the foetus embarks on further, complex rounds of differentiation of both embryonic and extra-embryonic tissues. Extensive descriptions of the developing embryonic features, organogenesis and early germ cell development can be found in Rugh (1968), Hogan *et al.* (1986) and Thieler (1989). Most of the developmental activity occurs before day 15 and the period that follows, up to birth at about day 19, is occupied by a growth phase during which the embryo effectively doubles in size.

5.2   TEST MATERIAL
5.2.1   Handling procedures

General advice on handling procedures, preparation and controls has been given in Chapter 1. Additional comments pertinent to germ cell tests are given here. When dosing animals, suitable respiratory protection is essential (the type of protection most suitable being determined by the physical characteristics of the test material). Clearly, exposure to test materials can come from the inhalation, dermal or even injection routes and suitable protective clothing as well as good safety practices are essential. Great care should be taken particularly when handling dusty solids, volatile liquids or gaseous materials. The risks for such test materials are clearly reduced by dissolving the test material in an inert solvent with a relatively high vapour pressure (e.g. water). The potential generation of aerosols and the hazards from animal excreta, bedding and carcasses should be considered.

All equipment contaminated with known genotoxic agents or materials of unknown toxicity should be thoroughly decontaminated using a strong cleansing agent, e.g. chloros, or should be destroyed by incineration.

5.2.2 Dose preparation

In the absence of stability data to the contrary, test material formulations should be prepared immediately prior to use. Several vehicles may have to be tested to find the most appropriate method of delivering the test material. In most cases, this is determined by the need to test at a maximum tolerated dose (MTD); determination of the MTD has recently been considered by an expert working party (Fielder *et al.*, in press).

It is essential that the vehicle does not adversely affect animals dosed with it, does not interfere with the objective of the study, and does not react with the test material. Dose volumes used should be compatible with the species being dosed, the identity of the vehicle and the route of exposure.

Ideally, the homogeneity and concentration of all preparations should be determined so that one may be confident that the desired dose is consistently administered. Although this is generally not conducted in short-term studies, it may be necessary when data are to be used for risk assessment. For inhalation studies, complicated and expensive atmosphere generation and analysis techniques may be required.

5.2.3 Control substances

5.2.3.1 *Negative (vehicle) controls*

Test protocols must include a group of animals treated with the vehicle control via the same route as used to administer the test material. The use of an untreated or negative control group in addition to the vehicle control group is considered unnecessary.

5.2.3.2 *Positive controls*

A positive control is used to demonstrate that the assay is functioning as expected. The dose of positive control administered should induce a borderline, but significant increase in chromosome anomalies thereby demonstrating the sensitivity of the assay. Where an assay is used regularly, and functions consistently within a laboratory, it should be possible to reduce the number of animals used as positive controls, e.g. in male germ cell tests, from five animals to two or three. Preston *et al.* (1981) list compounds that have proved positive in mammalian germ cell tests; of these substances, cyclophosphamide and mitomycin C are commonly chosen as positive controls.

Clearly, positive control materials must be safely handled as detailed in Section 5.2.1.

5.3   THE PROCEDURES
5.3.1   The test systems

The particular germ cell test chosen will be dictated by the purpose of the investigation; for example, in males, analysis of structural chromosome anomalies is generally undertaken in spermatogonia or primary spermatocytes; whereas screening for numerical chromosome anomalies is most appropriately carried out in metaphase II stage spermatocytes or in embryos.

5.3.1.1 Selection of the appropriate species and sex

Germ line tests are almost invariably carried out on rodent species and particularly the mouse. There are various reasons for this: mice are readily available commercially and are relatively inexpensive to purchase and maintain; the cytogenetics of this species has been widely investigated and described in the literature, and there is therefore considerable expertise in the various techniques upon which to draw.

Although the techniques discussed below were initially devised for experiments with the mouse, they are in principle equally applicable to other species. Indeed, many of them have been so used either directly or with some minor modifications.

It is recommended that males are used for the tests as preparation of male germ cells for microscopy is technically less difficult than for females. In addition, a substantially larger number of cells is available for analysis from each animal. One possible cautionary note, however, is the recent description of female-specific induction of dominant lethality in mice by selected compounds (discussed by Holmstrom, Palmer & Favor, 1992). The relative sensitivities of male and female germ cells to genotoxins is an area of uncertainty that is currently under active investigation.

5.3.1.2 Animal husbandry

The standard requirements of animal health and husbandry apply when using the germ cell methods. In brief, young, sexually mature animals will generally be used in the experiments. They must be healthy, allowed to acclimatise to their surroundings if purchased from a commercial supplier, maintained under optimal conditions of temperature and humidity with *ad lib* access to food and water, and handled in a manner that is as stress free as possible.

5.3.1.3 *Genetic stability*

The rate of *de novo* structural chromosome anomalies is very low in the mouse (Ford, 1970) and there is little reason to suspect that other laboratory species are any different. A check should be kept on this by comparing data from the vehicle control groups with the historical levels of aberrations in the laboratory. The frequency of spontaneous chromosome non-disjunction is known to be low in both male and female mammals of the common laboratory species (Mailhes, 1987). Any increase in the low spontaneous rate should be regarded as suspicious and provide grounds for reassessing or repeating the study.

5.3.1.4 *Tissue distribution*

It has been suggested that in the testis, germ cells, with the exception of spermatogonia, are effectively isolated from the general circulation via the so-called 'blood/testis' barrier (Setchell, 1978, 1980) or the Sertoli cell barrier (Russell, 1990). In the rat, germ cells beyond the spermatogonial stages of development lie within the Sertoli cell barrier (Russell, 1990). The implication of this is that compounds may have different abilities to reach target cells possibly depending on such factors as molecular size, lipid solubility, etc. Pharmacokinetic studies using radiolabelled compounds may show whether the test substance has the potential to reach target cells.

5.3.1.5 *Slide analysis*

The test systems involve the analysis of either mitotic or meiotic chromosomes and it is essential that all preparations are of good technical quality and are evaluated by trained and experienced investigators. Although some of the assays require a greater degree of cytogenetic expertise than for somatic tests such as the bone marrow method, acquisition of the necessary expertise is readily achieved and use of germ cell tests becomes relatively straightforward. All slides should be coded using a series of random numbers by an individual not subsequently involved in the chromosomal analysis. This code should not be broken until the study is complete. The vernier location of all aberrant cells (and preferably all cells analysed) should be recorded, the record of such analyses constituting the raw data of the study. All observations should therefore be fully described. Detailed descriptions of the types of and classifications of chromosomal aberrations is given by Savage (1976) and Scott *et al.* (1990) for mitotic chromosomes and by Searle (1975), Adler (1978 and

Cattanach (1982) for meiotic preparations. Illustrations of chromosome aberrations typically induced by genotoxins can be found in Adler (1982, 1984), Cattanach (1982), Jaquet and Pire (1984), Maihles, Yuan & Aardema (1990) and Rohrborn and Hansmann (1971).

5.3.1.6 *Administration of the test compound*

The route of administration of the test compound is dictated by the primary purpose of the study. Where information is to be generated for the purposes of risk assessment, the recommendation is that the compound is administered in a fashion that mimics potential human exposure. If, however, the study is initiated for hazard assessment, then the route of administration should be that which most effectively exposes the germ cell to the test compound, e.g. by intraperitoneal injection. The debate over the most suitable methods of administering test substances in genotoxicity studies has been summarised recently by Richold *et al.* (1990).

5.2.3   Male germ cells

The cytogenetic tests involving male germ cells have been widely used and consequently these assays are the most extensively validated. The endpoints that can be analysed are:

1. chromosome aberrations in mitotic, spermatogonial cells (Section 5.3.2.1);
2. reciprocal translocations (chromosome-type aberrations) at diakinesis/ metaphase I of meiosis to examine damage induced in the stem cell spermatogonia (Adler, 1974: Section 5.3.2.2);
3. chromatid-type aberrations at diakinesis/metaphase I to examine damage induced in primary spermatocytes (Adler, 1976; Walker, 1977: Section 5.3.2.2);
4. numerical chromosome anomalies at metaphase II (Brook & Chandley, 1986: Section 5.3.2.3).

The recommended method (detailed below) for preparation of spermatogonia and spermatocytes in the mouse is that of Evans, Breckon & Ford (1964). Breckon (1982) has discussed various slight modifications that may be necessary for optimising preparation quality in other rodent species. Various other methods have been described (Welshons, Gibson & Scandlyn, 1962; Meredith, 1969; Hoo & Bowles, 1971) however, they cannot be recommended as the preparation quality they produce is generally inferior to that of Evans *et al.* (1964) and moreover they may not provide a random sample of germ cells.

To carry out a germ cell assay in males, the animals are treated with the test material and are sampled at time(s) relevant to the germ cell stages being assessed. For spermatogonial cells it is necessary to treat the animals with a mitotic inhibitor such as colchicine 4 to 6 hours prior to sampling in order to accumulate sufficient numbers of cells for chromosomal analysis. A colchicine block is not recommended for spermatocyte preparations: such treatment may result in contraction of the bivalents to the extent that recognition of chromatid structure is hampered and identification of induced chromosome aberrations is hindered. At the appropriate sampling times the animals are killed and the testes are carefully dissected out. The germ cells are released by mechanical disruption of the tubules of the testes and the resultant cell suspension is treated with a hypotonic solution (1% trisodium citrate), fixed in 3:1 alcohol–acetic acid, dropped onto clean glass slides and air dried prior to staining and mounting (Evans *et al.*, 1964).

Due to the complexity and time consuming nature of the procedures involved in the preparation of germ cells for chromosomal analysis, it may be necessary to sub-divide an experiment into manageable replicates with at least one animal from each group in each replicate. If at all possible, however, all animals and cells should be handled and processed at the same time.

5.3.2.1 *Spermatogonia*

Chromosomal aberrations may be studied in the mitotically dividing spermatogonial cells undergoing differentiation in the testes. Chromatid-type aberrations must be analysed at the first mitotic division after treatment as they may be rapidly eliminated, e.g. due to cell death, and therefore not be detectable at subsequent divisions.

For the study of chromosomal aberrations in mitotically dividing spermatogonial cells, most protocols recommend a single administration at the MTD (see Fielder *et al.*, in press) to a group of five sexually mature males. Three sample times after dosing are used: usually 6 (or 12), 24 and 48 hours. In addition to the single dose/multiple sampling time protocol there are a number of multiple dose protocols. These are less favoured than the single dose protocol as repeated treatments may result in decreased aberration yields in spermatogonial cells due to cell death, increased compound elimination, adaptive metabolism or enhanced repair of lesions. In addition, repeated dosing is often more toxic so dose levels may have to be reduced. Five males per sampling interval should be used as vehicle controls. The positive control should also consist of five males, although as discussed earlier (Section 5.2.3.2) it may be possible to reduce this number.

The testes may be examined separately with 50 cells per testis being analysed but it is recommended that cells from both testes are pooled to obviate inter-testes variability in response, with 100 metaphases per animal being analysed.

If a positive result is obtained at the MTD, it may be considered necessary for risk assessment purposes to extend the study using several dose levels in order to elucidate a dose response

5.3.2.2 *Metaphase I stage spermatocytes*

Spermatogonial stem cells in mitotic metaphase cannot be distinguished from differentiating spermatogonia and so cannot be analysed directly; effects on this cell type can, however, be inferred through analysis of primary spermatocytes derived from treated stem cells. This will, however, only detect aberrations such as balanced translocations and certain inversions that are not lethal to the cell (Adler & Brewen, 1982). At diakinesis/ metaphase I of meiosis, reciprocal translocations induced in stem cells can be identified as they form characteristic ring or chain configurations. This assay can also be used to investigate damage induced in differentiating spermatogonia, although for these cell populations shorter intervals between treatment and sampling are necessary. Overall, three sampling times between 21 and 60 days post-dose are recommended to allow sampling of cells exposed as differentiating spermatogonia through to stem cells.

Chromosome damage induced in primary spermatocytes is analysed at multiple sampling times after dosing (Table 5.1) as the various stages of meiosis I possess variable sensitivity to genotoxins (Adler, 1977). The recommended protocol is a single MTD administration to five sexually mature males followed by multiple sampling times as detailed in Table 5.1. to screen different stages of germ cell development. As with spermatogonial studies, single dose/multiple sampling time studies are preferable to fractionated dose studies.

The testes may be examined separately with 50 cells per testis being analysed but, as with spermatogonia, it is recommended that the cells from both testes are pooled in case of inter-testes variability in response with 100 metaphases per animal being analysed. If a positive result is obtained, it may be considered necessary for risk assessment purposes to expand the study through use of several dose levels to investigate the possible dose–response.

5.3.2.3 *Metaphase II stage spermatocytes*

Metaphase II spermatocytes are used to assess the induction of non-disjunction in male germ cells (Allen *et al.*, 1986; Brook & Chandley, 1986). Although it is possible to analyse metaphase II spermatocytes for induced structural chromosome anomalies (Liang, Sherron & Johnston, 1986), the morphology of the chromosomes at this cell stage makes them unsuitable for routine analysis of chromosomal rearrangements. Aneuploidy is determined by counting chromosome numbers in the secondary spermatocytes. The

Table 5.1. *Germ cell stages sampled at different times after treatment (0 hours)*

Sampling time (post-dose)	Stage examined
24 hours	Diplotene at the time of dosing
5 days	Pachytene
9 days	Zygotene
11 days	Leptotene
12–14 days	Pre-leptotene

frequency of non-disjunction is best estimated by doubling the incidence of hyperhaploidy ($n + 1$); hypohaploidy ($n - 1$) tends to be an unreliable indicator due to possible confusion with artefactual loss of chromosomes during the processing of the cells. C-banding (Sumner, 1972), to demonstrate the pericentromeric heterochromatin, is an indispensable aid to unambiguous identification of hyperhaploid cells.

As the test compound may affect different stages of spermatogenesis, it may be necessary to use a number of sampling times. The intervals between dosing and sampling should take into account the possible influence of the test material on the rate of progression of cells through spermatogenesis and on stem cell toxicity (Liang & Pacchierotti, 1988). Autoradiographic studies can be used to determine the timing of spermatogenesis and to check for induced delays in cell cycle progression (Brook & Chandley, 1986). Cells can then be treated so as to expose various different stages of spermatogenesis and be sampled at the subsequent metaphase II stage of meiosis.

5.3.3   Female germ cells

The choice of cell stage to be analysed is largely dependent on the purpose of the investigation. The clastogenicity of a test compound may be examined using metaphase I stage oocytes. However, as the oocytes are treated when in the dictyate stage there is no DNA replication phase between exposure and analysis. Therefore, only S-independent compounds could reasonably be anticipated to show an effect at metaphase I (Brewen & Payne, 1976, 1978). If a compound is under test to determine its aneugenic potential, then analysis of metaphase II stage cells is appropriate.

In adult females, recommendation of intervals between treatment and sampling is problematical. The sensitivity of oocytes to mutagens is known to vary considerably during the period from the immature oocyte to that of a fully mature follicle. The US EPA Gene-Tox Program suggests intervals of 0.5, 6.5 and 28.5 days to encompass cells at different stages of development (Preston *et al.*, 1981). Whether use of all three intervals is either necessary or advisable is contentious (Albanese, 1987*a*).

In comparison to males, the number of germ cells available for analysis from each female is very small. Should a treatment also cause cell death, then the number of oocytes per female may be considerably reduced. Overall, it is much more convenient to think in terms of a total cell sample size rather than numbers of animals, although a minimum of ten females per treatment group is desirable. The number of cells obtained from each female will vary with strain and whether or not it has been exposed to a mutagen. Therefore the number of animals required may vary considerably from one study to another. A minimum of 150 cells per treatment group is recommended (Preston *et al.*, 1981).

5.3.3.1 *Metaphase I stage oocytes*

The recommended method for obtaining metaphase I oocytes is by induction of ovulation using exogenous gonadotrophic hormones and arrest of meiosis with colchicine (Brewen & Preston, 1982). The cells are then ovulated at the metaphase I stage rather than as normal at metaphase II. Less satisfactory, alternative methods for obtaining metaphase I oocytes are detailed in Tease and Cattanach (1986). Oocyte preparation for microscopy is carried out using the technique described by Tarkowski (1966). The metaphase I assay has been used in relatively few mutation experiments; critical reviews of published studies have been presented by Preston *et al.* (1981), Brewen and Preston (1982) and Adler and Brewen (1982).

5.3.3.2 *Metaphase II stage oocytes*

Cells at metaphase II are most easily obtained from females by hormonal induction of ovulation. The oocytes are ovulated at the metaphase II stage and can be collected from the oviduct and prepared for microscopy using the method described by Tarkowski (1966). This routine has been applied to the mouse (Hansmann & El-Nahass, 1979) and hamster species (Hansmann & Probeck, 1979).

Metaphase II oocytes are most appropriately used to determine whether a compound is capable of inducing non-disjunction in female germ cells. Aneuploidy is readily assessed through chromosome counts, although, because of the possibility of artefactual chromosome loss during cell preparation, only chromosome gains (hyperhaploidy) can be regarded as unambiguous evidence for chromosome non-disjunction. C-banding (Sumner, 1972), to demonstrate the pericentric heterochromatin, is an indispensable aid to accurate deter-mination of chromosome numbers. Although metaphase II oocytes can also be used to detect mutagen-induced chromosome structural damage, it is not recommended as a routine procedure. Studies investigating chemically induced aneuploidy in female germ cells have been critically reviewed by Mailhes, Preston and Lavappa (1986) and Tease and Cattanach (1986). In general, it has been found that oocytes treated within a few hours of ovulation are the most sensitive to the induction of chromosome non-disjunction.

5.3.4 Embryos

After exposure of parental germ cells to a test compound, either the pre- or post-implantation embryos that result from subsequent matings can be examined for chromosome damage. Since certain types of chromosome anomaly, e.g. monosomy, cause death of embryos before implantation, analysis of pre-implantation stages is generally more informative and therefore recommended.

5.3.4.1 Pre-implantation embryos

Pre-implantation embryos can be used to assess induced chromosome anomalies after exposure of either males or females. For mutagenicity screening, the most useful embryonic stage is the one-cell embryo (Tanaka, Katoh & Iwahana, 1981; Albanese, 1982, 1987*a*, *b*; O'Neill & Kaufman, 1987). One-cell embryos at metaphase of the first cleavage division can provide an assessment of the primary level of chromosome abnormalities, some of which may act as zygotic lethals or be indistinguishable at later embryonic stages. In addition, maternally and paternally derived chromosomes remain separate and can often be identified by their differing degrees of condensation; use of chromosome marker is advised, e.g. a Robertsonian metacentric chromosome, to identify one parental chromosome set and thereby reduce errors of identification.

Natural or gonadotrophin-induced ovulation may be used, although the latter will provide substantially more embryos per female. Various protocols are available for obtaining chromosome preparations from one-cell embryos: (i) *in vitro* fertilisation and culture of the eggs (Fraser & Maudlin, 1979); (ii) *in vivo* fertilisation followed by *in vitro* culture of the eggs (Fraser & Maudlin, 1979); (iii) *in vivo* fertilisation and development of the embryos (Maihles, Yuan & Aardema, 1990). The cells are generally prepared for microscopy using Tarkowski's (1966) method; more recently, Mikamo and Kamiguchi (1983) have described a technique which they suggest reduces cell breakage during preparation.

Dosed males can either be mated at weekly intervals over the whole of the spermatogenic cycle or during the post-meiotic stages which cover days 1 to 21 post-mating (Table 5.2). Where females are dosed, the same considerations apply as discussed in Section 5.3.3.

A minimum of 150 one-cell embryos per group should be scored using at least ten animals and, ideally, at least ten embryos should come from each female to give a representative sample. Both numerical and structural chromosome anomalies should be scored. Cells with loss of chromosomes resulting from technical artefacts of cell preparation should be excluded from the analysis. The types of structural chromosome aberrations that might be present will depend on the sex of the treated parent, the germ cell stage(s) exposed, and the compound under investigation (see Sections 5.3.2.2 and 5.3.3.1).

Later pre-implantation stage embryos, morulae and blastocysts are not recommended for mutagenicity screening, although they can provide information on the survival of chromosomally abnormal embryos (e.g. Hansmann, 1973).

5.3.4.2   *Post-implantation embryos*

Post-implantation embryos are not recommended for mutagenicity screening. They may be of value where information on the survival and development of chromosomally abnormal embryos is required. The small size and nature of embryos shortly after implantation (Hogan, Constantini & Lacy, 1986) make it difficult to obtain satisfactory chromosome preparations. From about day 10 p.c., chromosome preparations are more easily made. Chromosome preparations can be made from the whole embryo or from an organ such as the liver (Evans, 1987).

5.3.5   Heritable translocation test

Chromosome breakage in germ cells may give rise to balanced reciprocal translocations which, providing no loss of chromatin has occurred to make the rearrangement in a cell lethal, may be transmitted to the next generation. The frequency of translocation induction can be assessed in the primary spermatocytes of the treated animal but their heritability can only be inferred by reference to past studies in which directly estimated and transmitted frequencies have been compared (Ford *et al.*, 1969).

At the diakinesis/metaphase I stage of meiosis, most translocations form characteristic configurations, termed multivalents; the mechanics of formation and the typical features of these configurations have been reviewed (Searle, 1975; Adler, 1978; Cattanach, 1982). The two essential requirements for a multivalent to be produced are that the exchanged chromatin should pair during meiotic prophase and that a chiasma should form. If the exchanged segments are small resulting in failure of pairing or chiasma formation, the translocation will not be detected. It should be noted that, in addition to reciprocal translocations, other, rarer types of chromosome aberration can be

Table 5.2. *Germ cell stages sampled at different times after treatment*

Germ cells sampled	Interval (days)
Epididymal sperm	1–7
Testicular sperm and late spermatids	8–14
Early spermatids	15–21
Spermatocytes	22–35
Differentiating spermatogonia	36–49
Stem cell spermatogonia	>50

induced which can also form multivalents or unusual bivalents at diakinesis/metaphase I (see Evans, 1979; Cattanach, 1982).

Comprehensive descriptions of the procedure of a heritable translocation test have been given by Adler (1978, 1984) and Cattanach (1982). Although it is possible to screen for translocation induction in females (Searle & Beechey, 1974; Generoso *et al.*, 1978), almost invariably males are used. The males are dosed with the test compound and mated with untreated females either at specific intervals to investigate specific stages of spermatogenesis or continually to sample germ cells from the whole spermatogenic cycle (Table 5.2). The male offspring from these matings are then screened for the inheritance of translocations by fertility testing. Procedures for testing for translocations vary between laboratories: it can involve investigating numbers of live young, or the number of zygotic deaths at mid-gestation in females mated to F_1 males, or a combination of the two (Cattanach, 1982). The cytogenetic examination of the diakinesis/metaphase I stage of all the F_1 males, together with the chromosome banding of mitotic cells in the males lacking germ cells at this stage, would provide a 100% effective screen but is a time-consuming procedure.

The minimum number of F_1 males that should be tested is 400 (Generoso *et al.*, 1978); where cytogenetic analysis of diakinesis/metaphase I spermatocytes is undertaken, a sample of 25 cells is recommended as sufficient to determine whether or not an animal is a translocation carrier (Adler, 1978).

5.3.6 Tests under development

5.3.6.1 Synaptonemal complexes

Homologous chromosome pairing at pachytene of meiosis is mediated by a tripartite, proteinaceous structure called the synaptonemal complex (SC). It has been suggested that SC damage may provide a useful source of information on the effect of genotoxins on germ line cells (see Moses *et al.*, 1990; Allen *et al.*, 1990). SC preparations can be made from both male and female germ cells (Moses, 1977; Dresser & Moses, 1979; Mahadevaiah, Mittwoch & Moses, 1984). Analysis of these preparations, however, is carried out by electron microscopy and this cytogenetic approach therefore requires greater technical expertise than for the standard methods described above (Sections 5.3.2 and 5.3.3). Certain genotoxins have been shown to cause a variety of types of SC damage, but as many of these anomalies appear to be germ cell lethal events it has not yet proved possible to use this approach to quantify the likely impact of a compound on heritable genetic disease.

5.3.6.2 *Micronuclei in spermatids*

In essence, this method is an extension of the well-characterised micronucleus technique used in somatic cells. The micronuclei are screened in round, early spermatids following exposure of an earlier germ cell stage to the compound under investigation. This approach to germ cell study has been suggested to be technically easier than metaphase analysis. Unlike the somatic micronucleus assay, no recommended protocol is available and the method is unvalidated. There is no doubt, however, that germ cell exposure to mutagenic agents can result in an increased incidence of spermatids bearing micronuclei (Tates *et al.*, 1983; Toppari *et al.*, 1986).

5.3.6.3 *Non-isotopic* in situ *hybridisation*

Chromosome-specific DNA probes, labelled with reporter molecules such as biotin or digoxigenin, can be detected after *in situ* hybridisation using fluorescence microscopy or enzymatic reactions (Polak & McGee, 1990; Trask, 1991). The utility of nonisotopic *in situ* hybridisation (ISH) in mutation studies is under active investigation. ISH can be used to detect spontaneous chromosome anomalies, such as structural rearrangements (Cremer *et al.*, 1988; Ried *et al.*, 1992) and aneuploidy (Kuo *et al.*, 1991; Guttenbach & Schmid, 1991), and should have the potential to perform similar functions after mutagenic treatments of germ cells. The scope and limitations of this new technology will no doubt become much more clear once preliminary studies have been undertaken to determine its sensitivity in detecting and quantifying the effects of known genotoxins (Miller *et al.*, 1991; Salassidis *et al.*, 1992).

5.4   DATA PRESENTATION AND EVALUATION
5.4.1   Presentation of data

In addition to the general recommendations given in Chapter 1, it is essential that the following information is presented:

1. a full and accurate description of the test material and dose regimen;
2. the vehicle in which the test material was formulated and the stability and homogeneity of the formulation;
3. the genotype and husbandry of the animals;
4. complete and unambiguous presentation of the incidences of aberrations, from control and test groups, with clear classification of the different types: thus for structural anomalies as gaps, breaks and exchanges of both chromatid and chromosome type; and for numerical anomalies, as hypoploid, hyperploid and polyploid;
5. the types of statistical analysis used;
6. if transformed, derived or adjusted data is presented for the test material treated groups, a description of how this was carried out should be given.

Aberration data should be summarised in two ways: firstly, as frequency of each aberration type per cell; and secondly, as % aberrant cells.

5.4.2 Statistical analysis

The statistical analyses for germ cell tests are essentially identical to those for assays of chromosome aberration induction in somatic cells. Initially, if a compound has been given as a single dose, probably the MTD (Fielder *et al.*, in press), the frequency of chromosome anomalies in the treated group can be compared to the vehicle control using a non-parametric method, e.g. χ^2 or Fisher's exact test; this applies regardless of whether the endpoint is structural or numerical chromosome anomalies. Where more than one dose has been used, each individual dose can be compared to the vehicle control and, if appropriate, the data can also be analysed for a dose–response as discussed in detail in recent reviews (Lovell, 1989; Lovell *et al.*, 1989; Scott *et al.*, 1990). Professional advice should be sought where any uncertainty exists as to the appropriate way to analyse the data.

5.4.3 Repeat studies

Routinely, *in vivo* cytogenetic studies are conducted once. These studies are relatively expensive in time and resources and therefore they should be designed and conducted in such a way to produce a conclusive outcome. A repeat study may then only be justified if data are produced which are biologically suspicious without being statistically significant.

Clearly, the cause of an ambiguous outcome to a study needs to be identified and taken into consideration when contemplating a repeat experiment. Thought should also be given to the experimental design to modify any factors that might contribute to an unsatisfactory test, for example, increasing the numbers of cells if the analysis is marginal, or reconsideration of dose ranges and sampling intervals. Data from complementary studies may also provide relevant information or *in vivo* activity.

5.4.4   Interpretation of data

Germ cell cytogenetic tests are generally undertaken either for risk assessment or hazard assessment purposes. Only the heritable translocation assay provides data of direct relevance to the former objective. For the remaining tests, death of uncertain proportions of cells or embryos with induced chromosome anomalies makes it difficult to estimate, with any degree of confidence, the potential increment in induced heritable mutations after exposure to the test compound. The strength of these latter tests lies in their capacity to identify compounds with the ability to induce mutations in germ cells, i.e. hazard assessment.

Since the tests outlined in this chapter are not part of the initial screening programme for a test compound, their use implies a necessity to determine whether or not a compound is genotoxic in germ line cells. Identification of a positive result in such a study may therefore require that further information is obtained to allow risk estimates to be calculated. This subsequent step would involve either a heritable translocation test or a specific locus mutation experiment (Ehling, 1978; Searle, 1984). The observations in the original experiment are of value in determining the stages of germ cell development most susceptible to the genotoxic action of the compound.

If an experiment produces an ambiguous outcome, for example, an increase in the types of chromosome aberration associated with genotoxic activity but at an incidence that is not statistically significant, then consideration has to be given as to how to resolve this result. Various strategies are available, for example, increasing the size of the cell samples, choosing another route of administration of the compound, or adoption of an alternative germ cell assay.

5.5   SUMMARY

A wide range of cytogenetic assays is available to detect and quantify chromosome damage induced in mammalian germ cells. Of these assays, only those for spermatogonia and heritable translocations have regulatory guide-lines available (OECD, 1986). The lack of guidelines for the remaining assays reflects the fact that they do not play a role in the initial screening of novel or suspect compounds for genotoxicity. Rather, the principal function of these assays is to provide information on the potential of known genotoxins to induce heritable or potentially heritable genetic damage in germ cells. These assays are therefore only likely to be employed in those instances where there is a particular necessity to determine whether a genotoxic compound is active in germ cells.

5.6   REFERENCES

Adler, I.-D. (1974). Comparative cytogenetic study after treatment of mouse spermatogonia with mitomycin C. *Mutation Research*, **23**, 369–79

Adler, I.-D. (1976). Aberration induction by mitomycin C in early primary spermatocytes. *Mutation Research*, **35**, 247–56.

Adler, I.-D. (1977). Stage-sensitivity and dose–response study after irradiation of mouse primary spermatocytes. *International Journal of Radiation Biology*, **31**, 79–85.

Adler, I.-D. (1978). The cytogenetic heritable translocation test. *Biolisches Zentrablatt*, **97**, 441–51.

Adler, I.-D. (1982). Male germ cell cytogenetics. In *Cytogenetic Assays of Environmental Mutagens*, ed. T. C. Hsu, Allenheld Osmun, Totowa, NJ, pp. 249–76.

Adler, I.-D. (1984). Cytogenetic tests in mammals. In *Mutagenicity Testing: A Practical Approach*, ed. S. Venitt and J. M. Parry, IRL Press, Oxford, Washington, DC, pp. 275–306.

Adler, I.-D. & Brewen, J. G. (1982). Effects of chemicals on chromosome-aberration production in male and female germ cells. In *Chemical Mutagenesis: Principles and Methods for their Detection*, vol. 7, ed. F. J. de Serres and A. Hollaender, Plenum Press, pp. 1–35.

Albanese, R. (1982). The use of fertilised mouse eggs in detecting potential clastogens. *Mutation Research*, **97**, 315–26.

Albanese, R. (1987a). Induction and transmission of chemically induced chromosome aberrations in female germ cells. *Environmental and Molecular Mutagenesis*, **10**, 231–43.

Albanese, R. (1987b). Mammalian male germ cell cytogenetics. *Mutagenesis*, **2**, 79–85.

Allen, J. W., Liang, J. C., Carrano, A. V. & Preston, R. J. (1986). Review of literature on chemical-induced aneuploidy in mammalian male germ cells. *Mutation Research*, **167**, 123–37.

Allen, J. W., Poorman-Allen, P., Backer, L. C., Westbrook-Collins, B. & Moses, M. J. (1990). Synaptonemal complex analysis of mutagen effects on meiotic chromosome structure and behaviour. In *Banbury Report 34: Biology of Mammalian Germ Cell Mutagenesis*, eds. J. W. Allen, B. A. Bridges, M. F. Lyon, M. J. Moses and L. B. Russell, Cold Spring Harbor Press, pp. 155–69.

Beechey, C. V. & Searle, A. G. (1988). Effects of zero to four copies of chromosome 15 on mouse embryonic development. *Cytogenetics and Cell Genetics*, **47**, 66–71.

Breckon, G. (1982). A modified hypotonic treatment for increasing the frequency and quality of meiotic metaphases from spermatocytes of the Syrian hamster. *Stain Technology*, **57**, 349–54.

Brewen, J. G. & Payne, H. S. (1976). Studies on chemically induced dominant lethality. II. Cytogenetic studies of MMS-induced dominant lethality in maturing dictyate mouse oocytes. *Mutation Research*, **37**, 77–82.

Brewen, J. G. & Payne, H. S. (1978). Studies on chemically induced dominant lethality. III. Cytogenetic analysis of TEM-effects on maturing dictyate mouse oocytes. *Mutation Research*, **50**, 85–92.

Brewen, J. G. & Preston, R. J. (1982). Cytogenetic analysis of mammalian oocytes in mutagenicity studies. In *Cytogenetic Assays of Environmental Mutagens*, ed. T. C. Hsu, Allenheld Osmun, Totowa, NJ, pp. 277–87.

Brook, J. D. & Chandley, A. C. (1986). Testing for the chemical induction of aneuploidy in the male mouse. *Mutation Research*, **164**, 117–25.

Byskov, A. G. (1982). Primordial germ cells and regulation of meiosis. In *Germ Cells and Fertilization*, 2nd edn, eds. C. R. Austin and R. V. Short, Cambridge University Press, Cambridge, pp. 1–16.

Cattanach, B. M. (1982). The heritable translocation test in mice. In *Cytogenetic Assays of Environmental Mutagens*, ed. T. C. Hsu, Allenheld Osmun, Totowa, NJ, pp. 289–321.

Cremer, T., Lichter, P., Borden, J., Ward, D. C. & Manuelidis, L. (1988). Detections of chromosome aberrations in metaphase and interphase tumor cells by *in situ* hybridization using chromosome-specific library probes. *Human Genetics*, **40**, 235–46.

Dietrich, A. J. J. (1986). The influence of hypoxic treatment on the morphology of meiotic stages. II. Prophase of the first meiotic division of female mice up to dictyotene. *Genetica*, **70**, 161–5.

Dresser, M. E. & Moses, M. J. (1979). Silver staining of synaptonemal complexes in surface spreads for light and electron microscopy. *Experimental Cell Research*, **121**, 416–19.

Ehling, U. H. (1978). Specific-locus mutations in mice. In *Chemical Mutagens. Principles and Methods for their Detection*, vol. 5, eds. A. Hollaender & F. J. de Serres, Plenum Press, New York and London, pp. 233–56.

Evans, E. P. (1979). Cytological methods for the study of meiotic properties in mice. *Genetics*, **92**, 97–103.

Evans, E. P. (1987). Karyotyping and sexing of gametes, embryos and fetuses and in situ hybridization to chromosomes. In *Mammalian Development. A Practical Approach*, ed. M. Monk, IRL Press, Oxford, Washington, DC, pp. 93–114.

Evans, E. P., Breckon, G. & Ford, C. E. (1964). An air-drying method for meiotic preparations for mammalian testes. *Cytogenetics*, **3**, 289–94.

Fielder, R. J., Allen, J., Boobis, A., Botham P., Doe, J., Esdale, D., Gatehouse, D., Hodson-Walker, G., Morton, D., Kirkland, D. and Richold, M. (in press). Report of BTS/UKEMS Working Group on Dose Setting in *in vivo* Mutagenicity Tests.

Ford, C. E. (1970). The population genetics of other mammalian species. In *Human Population Cytogenetics*, eds. P. A. Jacobs, W. H. Price and P. Law, Edinburgh University Press, Edinburgh, pp. 229–39.

Ford, C. E., Searle, A. G., Evans, E. P. & West, B. J. (1969). Differential transmission of translocations induced in spermatogonia of mice by irradiation. *Cytogenetics*, **8**, 447–70.

Fraser, L. R. & Maudlin, I. (1979). Analysis of aneuploidy in first cleavage mouse embryos fertilized *in vitro* and *in vivo*. *Environmental Health Perspectives*, **31**, 141–9.

Generoso, W. M., Cain, K. T., Huff, S. W. & Gosslee, D. G. (1978). Heritable-translocation test in mice. In *Chemical Mutagens. Principles and Methods for their Detection*, vol. 5, eds. A. Hollaender and F. J. de Serres, Plenum Press, New York and London, pp. 55–77.

Guttenbach, M. & Schmid, M. (1991). Non-isotopic detection of chromosome 1 in human meiosis and demonstration of disomic sperm nuclei. *Human Genetics*, **87**, 261–5.

Hansmann, I. (1973). Induced chromosomal aberrations in pronuclei, 2-cell stages and morulae of mice. *Mutation Research*, **20**, 353–67.

Hansmann, I. & El Nahass, E. (1979). Incidence of nondisjunction in mouse oocytes. *Cytogenetics and Cell Genetics*, **24**, 115–21.

Hansmann, I. & Probeck, H. D. (1979). Chromosomal imbalance in ovulated oocytes from Syrian hamsters (*Mesocricetus auratus*) and Chinese hamsters (*Cricetulus griseus*). *Cytogenetics and Cell Genetics*, **23**, 70–6.

Hogan, B., Constantini, F. & Lacy, E. (1986). *Manipulating the Mouse Embryo. A Laboratory Manual.* Cold Spring Harbor Laboratory.

Holden, H. E. (1982). Comparison of somatic and germ cell models for cytogenetic screening. *Journal of Applied Toxicology*, **2**, 196–200.

Holmstrom, M., Palmer, T. & Favor, J. (1993). The rodent dominant lethal assay, this volume, Chapter 6.

Hoo, S. S. & Bowles, C. A. (1971). An air-drying method for preparing metaphase chromosomes from the spermatogonial cells of rats and mice. *Mutation Research*, **13**, 85–8.

Jaquet, P. & Pire, P. (1984). Morphological and cytogenetic studies of dominant lethality induced by mitomycin C and cyclophosphamide in female germ cells. The use of Robertsonian translocations as a 'marker system' to identify the zygote pronuclei. *Mutation Research*, **128**, 181–94.

Kuo, W.-L., Tenjin, H., Segraves, R., Pinkel, D., Golbus, M. S. & Gray, J. (1991). Detection of aneuploidy involving chromosomes 13, 18 or 21, by fluorescence *in situ* hybridisation (FISH) to interphase and metaphase amniocytes. *American Journal of Human Genetics*, **49**, 112–19.

Liang, J. C. & Pacchierotti, F. (1988). Cytogenetic investigation of chemically-induced aneuploidy in mouse spermatocytes. *Mutation Research*, **201**, 325–35.

Liang, J. C., Sherron, D. A. & Johnston, D. (1986). Lack of correlation between mutagen-induced chromosomal univalency and aneuploidy in mouse spermatocytes. *Mutation Research*, **163**, 285–97.

Lovell, D. P. (1989). Statistics and genetic toxicology – setting the scene. In *Statistical Evaluation of Mutagenicity Test Data*, ed. D. J. Kirkland, Cambridge University Press, Cambridge, New York, Port Chester, Melbourne, Sydney, pp. 1–25.

Lovell, D. P., Anderson, D., Albanese, R., Amphlett, G. E., Clare, G., Ferguson, R., Richold, M., Papworth, D. G. & Savage, J. R. K. (1989). Statistical analysis of *in vivo* cytogenetic assays. In *Statistical Evaluation of Mutagenicity Test Data*, ed. D. J. Kirkland, Cambridge University Press, Cambridge, New York, Port Chester, Melbourne, Sydney, pp. 184–232.

Mahadevaiah, S., Mittwoch, U. & Moses, M. J. (1984). Pachytene chromosomes in male and female mice heterozygous for the Is(7;1)40H insertion. *Chromosoma*, **90**, 163–9.

Mailhes, J. B. (1987). Incidence of aneuploidy in rodents. In *Aneuploidy, Part A: Incidence and Etiology*, eds. B. K. Vig and A. A. Sandberg, Alan R. Liss Inc., New York, pp. 67–101.

Mailhes, J. B., Preston, R. J. & Lavappa, K. S. (1986). Mammalian in vivo assays for aneuploidy in female germ cells. *Mutation Research*, **167**, 139–48.

Mailhes, J. B., Yuan, Z. P. & Aardema, M. J. (1990). Cytogenetic analysis of mouse oocytes and one-cell zygotes as a possible assay for heritable germ cell aneuploidy. *Mutation Research*, **242**, 89–100.

Meredith, R. (1969). A simple method for preparing meiotic chromosomes from mammalian testis. *Chromosoma*, **26**, 254–8.

Mikamo, K. & Kamiguchi, Y. (1983). A new assessment system for chromosomal mutagenicity using oocytes and early zygotes of the Chinese hamster. In *Radiation-Induced Chromosome Damage in Man*, eds. T. Ishihara and M. S. Sasaki, Alan R. Liss Inc., New York, pp. 411–32.

Miller, B. M., Zitzelberger, H. F., Weier, H.-Ul. G. & Adler, I.-D. (1991). Classification of micronuclei in murine erythrocytes: immunofluorescent staining using CREST antibodies compared to *in situ* hybridisation with biotinylated gamma satellite DNA. *Mutagenesis*, **6**, 297–302.

Monesi, V. (1962). Autoradiographic study of DNA synthesis and the cell cycle in spermatogonia and spermatocytes of mouse testis using tritiated thymidine. *Journal of Cell Biology*, **14**, 1–18.

Moses, M. J. (1977). Synaptonemal complex karyotyping in spermatocytes of the Chinese hamster (*Cricetulus griseus*). I. Morphology of the autosomal complement in spread preparations. *Chromosoma*, **60**, 99–125.

Moses, M. J., Poorman-Allen, P., Tepperberg, J. H., Gibson, J. B., Backer, L. C. & Allen, J. W. (1990). The synaptonemal complex as an indicator of induced chromosome damage. In *Banbury Report 34: Biology of Mammalian Germ Cell Mutagenesis*, ed. J. W. Allen, B. A. Bridges, M. F. Lyon, M. J. Moses and L. B. Russell, Cold Spring Harbor Press, pp. 133–53.

Oakberg, E. F. (1956). Duration of spermatogenesis in the mouse and timing of stages of the cycle of the seminiferous epithelium. *American Journal of Anatomy*, **99**, 507–16.

Oakberg, E. F. (1960). Mammalian gametogenesis and species comparisons in radiation response of the gonads. In *Effects of Radiation on Meiotic Systems*, IAEA, Vienna, pp. 3–15.

Oakberg, E. F. (1979). Timing of oocyte maturation in the mouse and its relevance to radiation-induced cell killing and mutational sensitivity. *Mutation Research*, **59**, 39–48.

Oakberg, E. F. (1981). The age at which the long-cycling spermatogonial stem-cell population is established in the mouse. In *Development and Function of the Reproductive Organs*, eds. A. G. Byskov and H. Peters, Excerpta Medica, Amsterdam, pp. 149–52.

OECD (1986). *OECD Guideline for Testing of Chemicals. Genetic Toxicology*, No. 483 & 485. Organisation for Economic Cooperation and Development, Paris, 23 October 1986.

O'Neill, G. T. & Kaufman, M. H. (1987). Cytogenetic analysis of first cleavage fertilized mouse eggs following in vivo exposure to ethanol shortly before and at the time of conception. *Development*, **100**, 441–8.

Peters, H. & McNatty, K. P. (1980). *The Ovary. A Correlation of Structure and Function in Mammals*, Granada Publishing, London, Toronto, Sydney, New York.

Preston, R. J., Au, W., Bender, M. A., Brewen, J. G., Carrano, A. V., Heddle, J. A., McFee, A. F., Wolff, S. & Wassom, J. S. (1981). Mammalian *in vivo* and *in vitro* cytogenetic assays: a report of the US EPA's Gene-Tox Program. *Mutation Research*, **87**, 143–88.

Polak, J. M. & McGee, J.O'D. eds. (1990). In Situ *Hybridisation. Principles and Practice*. Oxford University Press, Oxford, New York, Tokyo.

Richold, M., Ashby, J., Bootman, J., Chandley, A., Gatehouse, D. G. & Henderson, L. (1990). *In vivo* cytogenetic assays. In *Basic Mutagenicity Tests: UKEMS Recommended Procedures*, ed. D. J. Kirkland, Cambridge University Press, Cambridge, New York, Port Chester, Melbourne, Sydney, pp. 115–141.

Ried, T., Lengauer, C., Cremer, T., Wiegant, J., Raap, A. J., van der Ploeg, M., Groitl, P. & Lipp, M. (1992). Specific metaphase and interphase detection of the breakpoint in 8q24 of Burkitt lymphoma cells by triple-color fluorescence in situ hybridisation. *Genes, Chromosomes and Cancer*, **4**, 69–74.

Rohrborn, G. & Hansmann, I. (1971). Induced chromosome aberrations in unfertilized oocytes of mice. *Humangenetik*, **13**, 184–98.

Rugh, R. (1968). *The Mouse. Its Reproduction and Development.* Burgess Publishing Co., Minneapolis.

Russell, L. B. (1990). Barriers to entry of substances into seminiferous tubules: compatibility of morphological and physiological evidence. In *Banbury Report 34: Biology of Mammalian Germ Cell Mutagenesis*, eds. J. W. Allen, B. A. Bridges, M. F. Lyon, M. J. Moses and L. B. Russell, Cold Spring Harbor Laboratory Press, pp. 3–17.

Russell, L. B. & Shelby, M. D. (1985). Tests for heritable genetic damage and for evidence of gonadal exposure in mammals. *Mutation Research*, **154**, 69–84.

Salassidis, K., Huber, R., Zitzelberger, H. & Bauchinger, M. (1992). Centromere detection in vinblastine- and radiation-induced micronuclei of cytokinesis-blocked mouse cells by using *in situ* hybridisation with a mouse gamma (major) satellite DNA probe. *Environmental and Molecular Mutagenesis*, **19**, 1–6.

Savage, J. R. K. (1976). Classification and relationship of induced chromosomal structural changes. *Journal of Medical Genetics*, **13**, 103–22.

Scott, D., Danford, N. D., Dean, B. J. & Kirkland, D. J. (1990). Metaphase chromosome aberration assays *in vitro*. In *Basic Mutagenicity Tests: UKEMS Recommended Procedures*, ed. D. J. Kirkland, Cambridge University Press, Cambridge, New York, Port Chester, Melbourne, Sydney, pp. 62–86.

Searle, A. G. (1975). Radiation-induced chromosome damage and assessment of genetic risk. In *Modern Trends in Human Genetics*, ed. A. E. H. Emery, Butterworths, London, Boston, **2**, pp. 83–110.

Searle, A. G. (1984). The specific locus test in the mouse. In *Handbook of Mutagenicity Test Procedures*, 2nd edn, eds. B. J. Kilbey, M. Legator, W. Nichols and C. Ramel, Elsevier, Amsterdam, New York and London, pp. 373–91.

Searle, A. G. & Beechey, C. V. (1974). Cytogenetic effects of X-rays and fission neutrons in female mice. *Mutation Research*, **24**, 176–86.

Setchell, B. P. (1978). *The Mammalian Testis.* Paul Elek, London.

Setchell, B. P. (1980). The functional significance of the blood/testes barrier. *Journal of Andrology*, **1**, 3–10.

Speed, R. M. (1982). Meiosis in the foetal mouse ovary. I. An analysis at the light microscope level using surface spreading. *Chromosoma*, **85**, 427–37.

Sumner, A. T. (1972). A simple technique for demonstrating centromeric heterochromatin. *Experimental Cell Research*, **75**, 304–6.

Tanaka, N., Katoh, M. & Iwahana, S. (1981). Formation of chromosome-type aberrations at the first cleavage after MMS treatment in late spermatids of mice. *Cytogenetics and Cell Genetics*, **31**, 145–52.

Tarkowski, A. K. (1966). An air-drying method for chromosome preparation from mouse eggs. *Cytogenetics*, **5**, 394–400.

Tates, A. D., Dietrich, A. J. J., de Vogel, N., Neuteboom, I. & Bos, A. (1983). A micronucleus method for detection of meiotic micronuclei in male germ cells of mammals. *Mutation Research*, **121**, 131–8.

Tease, C. & Cattanach, B. M. (1986). Mammalian cytogenetic and genetic tests for non-disjunction. In *Chemical Mutagens, Principles and Methods for their Detection*, vol. 10, ed. F. J. de Serres, Plenum Press, New York, London, pp. 215–83.

Thieler, K. (1989). *The House Mouse. Atlas of Embryonic Development.* Springer-Verlag, Berlin, Heidelberg, New York.

Toppari, J., Lahdetie, J., Harkonen, P., Eerola, E. & Parvinen, M. (1986). Mutagen effects on rat seminiferous tubules in vitro: induction of meiotic micronuclei by adriamycin. *Mutation Research*, **171**, 149–56.

Trask, B. J. (1991). Fluorescence *in situ* hybridisation. *Trends in Genetics*, **7**, 149–54.

Walker, H. C. (1977). Comparative sensitivities of meiotic prophase stages in male mice to chromosome damage by acute X- and chronic gamma irradiation. *Mutation Research*, **44**, 427–32.

Welshons, W. J., Gibson, B. H. & Scandlyn, B. J. (1962). Slide processing for the examination of male mammalian meiotic chromosomes. *Stain Technology*, **37**, 1–5.

6

The rodent dominant lethal assay

L. M. Holmstrom   A. K. Palmer   J. Favor

6.1   INTRODUCTION

The rodent dominant lethal test is used, in a strategic sense, to determine whether a substance which is genotoxic in somatic cells is also genotoxic in germ cells. The test therefore assesses the ability of an agent to reach the gonads and gametes and induce lesions which, when expressed in the fertilised egg, cause premature death of the developing embryo (Anderson, Bateman & McGregor, 1983; Green *et al.*, 1985). If embryonic development is stopped, following fertilisation but prior to implantation of the egg in the uterine wall, the event is a *pre-implantation loss*. If, on the other hand, developmental arrest and embryo death takes place at a later stage in pregnancy, the event represents a *post-implantation loss* (Bateman, 1958).

Post-implantation losses can be sub-divided into early and late deaths. These can be induced at any time from conception through birth, although early deaths predominate to the extent that they have been considered most indicative of a dominant lethal effect (Favor, Soares & Crenshaw, 1978). Late embryonic deaths may also be caused by a greater number of confounding factors including adverse environmental conditions such as nutritional deprivation, oxygen starvation and microbial infections (Bateman, 1958; Röhrborn, 1968).

Dominant lethal tests can be conducted in both male and female animals, although males have traditionally been investigated (Sudman & Generoso, 1991). Mice and rats are normally favoured although less commonly used species such as the hamster and the guinea pig have also been studied (Lyon & Smith, 1971). Whatever the species or sex tested, the basis of the assay remains the same. First, exposure of the animals to the test agent, be it chemical, physical or viral (Epstein & Shafner, 1968; Reddi & Vasudevan, 1968; Pathki & Polasa, 1988); secondly, mating of the treated animals to untreated animals of the opposite sex; and thirdly, examination of pregnant females to assess the frequency of live and dead implants among the offspring.

The study of exposed males rather than females is primarily due to the inherent limitations of the female-based assay. These include 1) difficulty in separating treatment-related genotoxic effects from physiological variables such as hormonal status or uterine damage affecting survival of implants; 2) difficulty in distinguishing between toxic and genotoxic responses in the event of extensive oocyte killing; 3) inability to assess exposed and mated females more than once (Maxwell & Newell, 1973; Verschaeve and Léonard, 1984; Mattison & Thomford, 1989).

The rodent dominant lethal test provides general information on the potential of an agent to interfere with critical hormonal, metabolic or genetic processes in the gonads. Induction of dominant lethals, therefore, is part of a spectrum of germ cell effects which include impaired fertility or sterility, pre-implantation and post-implantation embryo losses, as well as growth of genetically, morphologically and behaviourally abnormal offspring (Trasler *et al.*, 1986; Anderson *et al.*, 1987; Au *et al.*, 1990).

Dominant lethal effects are known to arise from gross cytogenetic disturbances, including chromosomal deletions, rearrangements, monosomies and trisomies (Matter & Jaeger, 1975; Hitotsumachi & Kikuchi, 1977; Russell *et al.*, 1989). A role for point mutations in the aetiology of dominant lethality is also possible (Propping, Röhrborn & Buselmaier, 1972; Nagao, 1988). However, non-genetic mechanisms such as gonadal toxicity, DNA methylation disturbances and hormonal imbalances may also play a part in the induction of dominant lethality (Chellman, Bus & Working, 1986; Holliday, 1987; Working, 1989).

If the metabolism of the test material is similar in rodents and man, positive dominant lethal findings imply a potential risk to human germ cells (Rhomberg *et al.*, 1990). Follow-up studies may be conducted on such compounds to characterise the particular lesion underlying dominant lethal induction. Toxicologically, the nature, degree and stage specificity of the gonadal damage can be examined through reproductive studies and histopathological analysis (Hardin, 1983; McGregor *et al.*, 1983; Lee & Kinney, 1989). Genetically, the level of transmitted heritable mutations may be assessed via use of specific locus, heritable translocation, dominant cataract or enzyme activity tests (Russell & Shelby, 1985; Generoso *et al.*, 1990; Favor, 1990). However, such tests that use large numbers of animals must be carefully justified, and alternative approaches may be considered (Adler & Brewen, 1982).

As a test for the genotoxic effects on germ cells, the dominant lethal assay should be used only when positive *in vivo* findings from short-term mutagenicity studies, e.g. micronucleus, sister chromatid exchange or DNA strand break and repair tests, indicate that a compound is potentially harmful to mammalian germ cells. As such, the rodent dominant lethal test is part of a hierarchical testing strategy which begins with the application of *in vitro* mutagenicity assays and may culminate with the use of the above described large-scale animal tests for examining heritability of genetic defects (Holden, 1982; Ashby, 1986; Arni *et al.*, 1988; DH, 1989).

Given prior evidence of somatic genotoxicity, a positive dominant lethal effect implies that the test compound is a germ cell genotoxin in the species, strain and sex used. A negative dominant lethal response indicates either no gonadal genotoxicity or unsuitability of the test system to evaluate a particular germ cell effect (Adler & El Tarras, 1990; Katoh *et al.*, 1990; Mailhes & Aardema, 1992).

6.2   TEST CONDUCT

The rodent dominant lethal test can be conducted using a variety of dosing and mating regimens. Before performing a test, it is essential that the magnitude of the expected dominant lethal effect is considered with respect to available genotoxicity data. This is important because rodent males can often sire normal litters in spite of marked testicular damage or an impairment of spermatogenesis. The biological background, as well as advantages and disadvantages of a given study design, are further discussed below.

6.2.1   Dominant lethal tests in males

Mammalian spermatogenesis can be divided into three distinct phases. In the first phase, spermatogonial stem cells proliferate to produce spermatocytes whilst maintaining their cell number by renewal; in the second phase, the spermatocytes undergo reductional division during meiosis to produce haploid spermatids; and in the third phase, the spermatids develop via gradual and complex biochemical and morphological processes into mature spermatozoa (Clermont, 1972; Amann, 1989; Erickson, 1990).

Based on morphology, the first and third phases of spermatogenesis show species-specific features, while spermatocytes throughout meiosis present similar morphology in distinct mammalian species (Clermont, 1972). Considerable species-related differences, notably between rodents and man, appear to exist in the capacity for stem cell regeneration and repopulation of the seminiferous epithelium (Meistrich, 1986). Each cell type is also characterised throughout spermatogenesis by its own metabolic activity, DNA repair capacity and higher order chromosomal organisation. Together, these properties modulate the susceptibility of the germ cells towards genotoxic challenges (Lee, 1983).

In mice, spermatogenesis, from stem cell spermatogonia to mature epididymal sperm, lasts 42 days; in rats, around 63 days. The developmental stages for rats and mice subdivide as in Table 6.1 (Leblond & Clermont, 1952; Oakberg, 1956; Fox & Fox, 1967).

Table 6.1.

Spermatogenic cell stage	Duration in days	
	Mouse	Rat
Differentiating spermatogonia	6	4.5
Differentiating spermatocytes	14	10.5
Differentiating spermatids	9	11
Testicular spermatozoa	5.5	22*
Epididymal spermatozoa	7.5	15
All germ cell stages combined	42	64*

*Duration may vary between different rat strains (Clermont, 1972).

In a typical dominant lethal test, male mice or rats are given a single, or 2–5 daily, doses of the test material, then mated with successive groups of virgin females for a specific length of time. These sequential matings attempt to sample exposed germ cells from different stages of spermatogenesis, notably the most sensitive stages of gamete development (Ehling, 1977; Shelby *et al.*, 1986). The frequent choice of subacute, in preference to acute, dosing, is probably based on the experiences of individual laboratories using the two approaches. Thus many compounds appear to induce higher levels of dominant lethals when given as fractionated doses over 2–5 days, compared with an equivalent or near equivalent total dose given only once (Green *et al.*, 1973; Shelby *et al.*, 1986; Ehling & Neuhäuser-Klaus, 1990).

The shorter the interval between each mating occasion, the greater the chances are of identifying stage(s) of spermatogenesis sensitive to potential dominant lethal induction. The choice of mating intervals, whether 7 day, 4 day or even shorter, should therefore be dictated by considering all relevant study aspects, including the sensitivity of the test system, available reproductive data and any constraints on the numbers of animals to be used.

6.2.2   Dominant lethal tests in females

Oogenesis in mammals is composed of three distinct phases involving proliferation, growth and maturation of the germ cells. Stem cells derive from primordial germ cells which originate in the yolk sac epithelium, after which they migrate to the gonads on days 9–12 of embryo development where they differentiate into oogonia (Kuhlmann, 1970). Oogonia then proliferate and divide by mitosis to form a reservoir of primary oocytes. In the growth phase, these produce large amounts of messenger RNA, as well as ribosomal RNA and proteins which are required during the early phases of embryo development. In the subsequent maturation process, meiosis occurs during which the diploid oocytes undergo a reduction in chromosome number to give a haploid egg.

In mice and rats, the prophase stages of meiosis occur virtually synchronously before birth, starting around day 13 of intra-uterine life. The chromosomes remain arrested in an extended diplotene stage of meiosis until ovulation and fertilisation occurs. Throughout this period, the oocyte chromosomes have a highly elongated, diffuse appearance (Kuhlmann, 1970).

In female dominant lethal experiments, the duration of dosing and mating procedure adopted is similar to those used in the male-based assay (Hess, 1973; Badr & Badr, 1974; Röhrborn & Hansmann, 1974). In females, a conventional dosing period will only give rise to dominant lethals which are derived from lesions induced in the maturing dictyate oocyte (Brewen & Payne, 1976; Generoso *et al.*, 1989*a*). Other testing strategies are, therefore, required to study compound interferences with the earlier stages of oocyte development (Hansmann, 1974; Verschaeve and Léonard, 1984). It should also be noted that compounds which induce embryo lethals primarily via chromosome non-disjunction may require careful study design in the female dominant lethal test (Röhrborn & Hansmann, 1974; Generoso *et al.*, 1989*a*).

Confirmation of the genetic nature of dominant lethals in females should be sought to evaluate the possible contributory role of maternal toxicity in any germ cell effect. Cytogenetic techniques are often used and involve the collection and chromosomal analysis of spontaneously and synchronously ovulated, or hormonally induced superovulated oocytes from the treated females (Hess, 1973; Hansmann, 1974; Brewen & Payne, 1976). Another procedure aimed at excluding maternal toxicity as the cause for dominant lethal induction is to transfer zygotes deriving from exposed oocytes into treated and control treated foster mothers and allow them to develop until assessment. Any dominant lethal effect is confirmed by aberration analysis of first-cleavage mitotic chromosomes in zygotes collected from separately treated females (Katoh *et al.*, 1990; Sudman & Generoso, 1991).

6.2.3   Dominant lethal tests with sub-chronic treatments

Dominant lethal assays using sub-chronic treatments over a prolonged period to assess for potential cumulative damage to the germ cells are occasionally performed (Generoso *et al.*, 1983; Trasler, Hales & Robaire, 1986; Grahn, Carnes & Farrington, 1986). There are, however, two main disadvantages with such sub-chronic studies. First, they provide no indication of the particular germ cell targeted; secondly, the doses used may have to be very low due to general toxic side effects to the animals. Sub-chronic treatment may also affect animal fertility and cell maturation leading to difficulties in assessment. Furthermore, if the germ cell stage, specifically sensitive to the genotoxic effect, is of short duration, an increase in dominant lethals may not be demonstrable over the experimental period due to dilution of damage or induction of adaptive DNA repair processes (Lee, 1983).

On the contrary, there is evidence that chronic low doses of strong geno-toxins may in some cases be more potent than much higher single doses with regards to inducing dominant lethality (Epstein *et al.*, 1970; Sheu & Moreland, 1983; Generoso *et al.*, 1983). A case can therefore be made for sub-chronic dominant lethal tests under certain circumstances, especially where animal conservation is important. Thus, a routine dominant lethal test may use more than 1000 animals, while a sub-chronic study requires only a fraction of that number.

In a sub-chronic dominant lethal test, male mice are commonly dosed for 6–8 weeks and rats for 8–10 weeks prior to mating to cover the duration of spermatogenesis. However, since ultimately all agents which induce dominant lethals do so by interfering with the meiotic or post-meiotic stages of sperm development, a shorter dosing period may be scientifically and practically justified if the specific aim of the study is to detect, rather than characterise, a potential dominant lethal effect.

6.3   CRITICAL FACTORS
6.3.1   Animals
6.3.1.1   *Species variations*
Species differences in agent-induced germ cell toxicity and genotoxicity have been demonstrated in many assays, including the rodent dominant lethal test (Lyon & Smith, 1971). The reasons for species variation in responsiveness are clearly complex and cover pharmacokinetic, metabolic, physiological and DNA repair-related functions (Lee, 1983; Generoso, Cain & Hughes, 1985). Choice of species for dominant lethal testing should therefore always be dictated by any previous information regarding species sensitivity and the objectives of the study. Where human risk assessment is concerned, it is desirable to use the species which most closely resembles man as regards metabolism of the test substance (Roberts *et al.*, 1989).

6.1.3.2   *Strain variations*
Rodent strains may vary in their susceptibility to dominant lethal induction (Léonard *et al.*, 1972; Shelby *et al.*, 1986; Lovell, Anderson & Jenkinson, 1987). In rare cases, such variations may give rise to qualitative differences in dominant lethal induction apparently due to the strain-dependent repair capacity which fertilised eggs demonstrate (Röhrborn & Hansmann, 1974; Brandriff & Pedersen, 1981; Sheu & Moreland, 1983). It is therefore

important that the strain selected for dominant lethal testing is of proven fecundity, and has a low spontaneous rate of embryonic death with no known DNA repair defect (Epstein *et al.*, 1972; Lovell *et al.*, 1987).

Outbred rodent strains or F_1 hybrids should preferably be used, as these normally perform better in terms of high pregnancy and low spontaneous dominant lethal mutations. Mouse strains carrying t-lethals, translocations or similar cytogenetic abnormalities should not be used in routine dominant lethal screens. Ideally, the normal pregnancy rate for the mouse strain used should exceed 80% while the regular litter size should be greater than ten live implants per dam. The proportion of animals with more than two early deaths should be as low as possible and average no more than 10% within the negative control group.

6.3.1.3 Sex differences

Quantitative, as well as qualitative sex differences in dominant lethal testing have been reported (Generoso *et al.*, 1983; Katoh *et al.*, 1990). Such sex-related responses have been attributed to the chromosomal condensation states of the germ cells. As a consequence, reactive agents may have differential access to DNA or other critical cellular targets in germ cells of the two sexes (Katoh *et al.*, 1990; Sudman & Generoso, 1991). Other factors may, however, also be involved in such sex-dependent dominant lethal induction (Oakberg, 1979; Mattison & Thomford, 1989).

6.3.1.4 Animal source and age

Rodents should be obtained from recognised suppliers to minimise heterogeneity between animals and ensure that an acceptable breeding performance is established. If in-house stock colonies are used, important variables such as fecundity and spontaneous frequencies of dominant lethality should be fully evaluated before testing. Historical records should be kept of animal responses and any unusual variations documented (Röhrborn, 1968; Ray & Hyneck, 1973).

Young, sexually mature, adult male and female rodents should be used for dominant lethal testing, as age may affect responsiveness (Searle & Beechey, 1985). Typical age ranges are 8–10 weeks for male and 6–8 weeks for female mice. For rats, 10–12 weeks for males and 8–10 weeks for females are more common. The weight and age of each successive batch of females should be the same, where possible.

6.3.1.5 Number of animals

In a rodent dominant lethal test using males, the number of animals exposed per group should be dictated by the objectives of the study and the assurance required to discriminate between a positive and negative effect. Obviously, fewer males are required to demonstrate a response to a potent as opposed to a weak germ cell genotoxin. For practical reasons, 15–20 treated males are often recommended per treatment or vehicle control group, although smaller numbers can be used in positive control groups (see below). Male to female mating ratios of 1:2 or 1:3 are frequently used for males of high fecundity, while a ratio of 1:1 may be more suitable for less fertile males. In the latter case, a larger number of males should be treated to give a sufficient number of pregnant females for analysis (Ray & Hyneck, 1973; Dean & Johnstone, 1977; Ehling *et al.*, 1978).

Since the male is the experimental unit in dominant lethal testing, one disadvantage with unequal mating ratios is that the statistical analysis becomes more complicated. Where the main study objective is to characterise or confirm a weak dominant lethal effect, a 1:1 mating ratio using a large number of treated males, e.g. 40, may, therefore, be the simplest approach (Chanter *et al.*, 1989; Ehling & Neuhäuser-Klaus, 1989).

The inclusion of a positive control group in dominant lethal testing is a matter of ethical debate. When a laboratory has extensive experience of testing and sufficient background data, the routine use of a positive control group may not be necessary. However, when a dominant lethal test is developed or a new rodent species or strain obtained, the addition of a positive control group to the study is recommended. The number of positive control animals used should be as low as possible; a typical number of treated males is 10. A reduced period of mating using the most sensitive period of gametogenesis is acceptable, where the effect of a control agent is well known. Stage-specific effects in germ cells exposed to genotoxins have been described by Fox & Fox (1967), Röhrborn (1970), Ehling (1977), Lyon (1981) and Adler & Brewen (1982).

6.3.2   Test materials

General information on test materials has been given in Chapter 1.

The dominant lethal test is normally used as a screen for potential germ cell effects following observations made in somatic assays. As a result, considerable information concerning the properties, solubility and stability of the test material under defined conditions often exists. Such data should be reviewed carefully before testing to identify potential problems associated with dose formulation, administration and toxicity (Ray & Hyneck, 1973).

6.3.2.1 Dose preparation

All test materials of chemical or biological origin should be freshly prepared on the day of dosing and analysed routinely with respect to stability, concentration and homogeneity as appropriate.

6.3.2.2 Vehicle controls

The solvent used should not adversely affect the physiology of the animal. For water miscible materials, distilled water or isotonic saline is appropriate. Hydrophobic substances can be prepared in corn oil, gum arabic or 0.5% (w/v) carboxymethoxycellulose with the optional addition of a small amount of Tween 80 as a wetting agent. Homogenisation or emulsification of insoluble materials may in some instances become necessary (Ashby, 1987; Paolini, Biagli & Forti, 1988). The procedure for preparing the vehicle control should, as far as possible, follow the method used to dissolve or suspend the test substance.

There is evidence that solvent–drug interactions may occur in the course of *in vivo* genotoxicity testing (Wallig *et al.*, 1989; Simula & Priestly, 1991). It may, therefore, be advisable to include a further, untreated control group of animals to assess the possible effects contributed by unusual or potentially active vehicles in any dominant lethal response (Generoso *et al.*, 1984).

6.3.2.3 Positive controls

It may be desirable to include a defined low dose of a documented dominant lethal-inducing chemical as a positive control substance (Section 6.3.1.5). Examples of commonly used positive controls, including recommended dose levels have been described (Brewen & Payne, 1976; Ehling, 1977; Dean, Anderson & Srám, 1981). A compilation of substances tested as positive in the rodent dominant lethal assay can be found in Green *et al.* (1985).

When selecting positive control dose levels, especially during subacute and chronic testing, the following factors should be considered: 1) dose elimination or dose interaction may lead to decreased or increased responses; 2) adaptive metabolic or DNA repair processes may reduce the rate of death; 3) animal genotype may influence the frequency of dominant lethality (Lee, 1983; Shelby *et al.*, 1986). It is, for these reasons, recommended that a pilot study is performed when a dominant lethal assay is being developed in a laboratory so that the relative induction of lethals by a specific control agent is known.

The nature of the test material and its vehicle may be relevant to the selection of positive controls. Typical water-based controls are cyclophosphamide and various alkyl methanesulphonates (Ehling, 1977; Dean *et al.*, 1981). Chlorambucil provides an example of a hydrophobic positive control substance (Russell *et al.*, 1989).

6.3.2.4 Reference substances

Occasionally, it may be appropriate to use chemicals, structurally and/or functionally related to the test material. Such reference substances can be tested instead of, or in addition to, the positive control substance. The same criteria should apply to both test substance and reference material, e.g. as regards levels of toxicity induced (Saito-Suzuki, Teramoto & Shirasu, 1982; Shelby *et al.*, 1986; Working *et al.*, 1987).

6.3.2.5   *Route of administration*

The dominant lethal test can be conducted using a variety of dose routes. Choice of dose route can be based on different considerations. For hazard identification of compounds showing good absorption, oral dosing is normally preferred. Appropriate parenteral dose routes may, however, also be used to evaluate compounds which do not require bioconversion in the liver or gut. For risk assessment purposes, the dose route may also be dictated by the specific need to mimic the actual human exposure situation, in which case the most common route of exposure should be chosen.

In the absence of such expressed objectives, it is recommended that readily soluble test substances are given as intraperitoneal (i.p.) injections. This follows because many chemicals are more toxic and genotoxic to the germ cells when given i.p. compared to orally (Soares & Sheridan, 1977; Sỳkora, 1981; Mailhes, Yuan & Aardema, 1990). Qualitative differences where i.p., but not oral dosing induced a dominant lethal effect have been reported (Shibuya, Mijamae & Murota, 1988).

In general, it is recommended that poorly soluble test substances or suspensions are examined with respect to absorption from the application site, as failure to do so may invalidate the study objectives. Such information on compound absorption is readily gained from gross post-mortem examinations of a small group of animals, treated with the highest test dose to be used.

6.3.2.6   *Selection of dose levels*

Non-toxic substances should be tested to a fixed limit dose in line with the norm for other somatic *in vivo* assays. Recent revisions of EEC guidelines for toxicity and genotoxicity testing stipulate maximum doses of 2 g/kg for single and 1 g/kg for repeated treatments (EEC, in press). This Working Group recommends that these limit doses should also apply to dominant lethal testing, unless there are compelling reasons for using higher exposure levels.

Where reliable toxicity information on a test substance is available, it is usually sufficient to perform a limited toxicity test using a small number of animals. The objective of such testing is to identify suitable dose levels for the dominant lethal test in a given species, strain and sex, following the chosen route of administration. For compounds of unknown toxicity, it is recommended that a more detailed toxicity study is undertaken. In both cases, any compound effect on the fecundity of the exposed animals should ideally be considered (Section 6.4.6).

Various toxicological methods to set doses for short term animal geno-toxicity assays have been described (De Pass, 1989). Such approaches usually aim to determine a maximum tolerated dose, e.g. as defined by body weight loss, adverse clinical signs in living animals or gross post mortem findings, in the absence of treatment-related deaths (Thompson & Gibson, 1984; Van den Heuvel *et al.*, 1990; Mackay & Elliott, 1992; Fielder *et al.*, 1992).

During sub-chronic dominant lethal tests, it is important that persistent body weight loss is avoided. Instead, a minor reduction in body weight gain at the highest compound dose should be aimed for (Khera *et al.*, 1976).

The number of test groups for the evaluation of potential dominant lethal effects should always reflect the objectives of the study. For routine screening purposes, three groups are typically used. The highest test dose should be one which induces evident toxicity. Lower doses can be set at halving or half-logarithmic proportions of this dose. However, the number of dose groups, dosages and dosing intervals should always be decided on a case by case basis.

6.3.2.7 *Setting of dose volumes*

Two common methods for dose volume setting exist. The first procedure relies on adjustments of a pre-determined dose volume, e.g. 10 ml/kg, in accordance with the weight of the test animal. The second uses a fixed dose, e.g. 0.1 ml, given to young adult mice of a pre-determined weight range (Bishop *et al.*, 1983).

Common p.o. application volumes are 5, 10 or 20 ml/kg body weight. Occasionally, dose volumes of 25 ml/kg or 30 ml/kg may be justified if a higher dose is required for agents with hydrophobic properties and limited solubility. Agents administered via parenteral routes should be given in dose volumes which minimise physical stress to the animal, e.g. 5 ml/kg body weight in the case of i.p. dosing. As a rule, the lowest amount of solvent compatible with the test material and the physiological space available in the animal should apply.

6.4 ANIMAL HUSBANDRY
6.4.1 Housing and management

Animal acclimatisation, housing and management routines should conform to accepted principles and procedures for the handling of laboratory rodents (UFAW, 1987; HMSO, 1990).

6.4.2 Mating procedure

It is important to know that mating has occurred to exclude the possibility that the libido or fertility of an animal has been affected by a treatment (Lane *et al.*, 1985). In mice, confirmation of mating is accomplished via vaginal plug examination; in rats via vaginal plug or smear analysis. A smear analysis is only required when no plug exists, in which case presence of sperm provides proof of mating. Determination of the date of conception enables all pregnant females to be assessed in the same stage of pregnancy.

Following sub-chronic animal exposures, confirmation of matings via the above procedures is essential. If a female is found to be non-pregnant following the first co-housing period, a second mating can be performed with fresh females to maximise the number of pregnancies. It also helps to identify whether the failure of conception was treatment related and whether the dominant lethal effect is reversible (Tariq *et al.*, 1990).

6.4.3   Identification and markings

Animals should be identified uniquely via ear punching or other permanent marker systems. Ear tags are not recommended as these may get torn off and cause septicaemias.

Mating and killing records should be such that each mating is uniquely identified, by animal or cage number, until assessment.

6.4.4   Randomisation systems

Before randomisation, obvious sources of animal variation should be eliminated as far as possible. This is ensured by ordering animals from suppliers to specified criteria regarding species, strain, weight, age and clinical condition. Animals of suspect health or unusual weight should not be used.

Identifiable sources of variation that cannot be eliminated should be distributed equally across control and test groups. For example, siblings should be allocated evenly to the various dose groups (Chanter *et al.*, 1989). Following these initial measures, randomisation procedures for allocation of animals to dose groups should be applied as a final step to equalise any remaining variance. This procedure is suitably accomplished via the use of a stratified randomisation process.

Each animal cage should be distributed on the rack so as to equalise potential environmental influences (light, temperature, humidity) across the dose groups. An organised or structural distribution of the cages, e.g. via sequential group randomisations or Latin square designs is preferable as it facilitates the tasks of dosing and handling and reduces the scope for human error.

6.4.5   Animal observation

All animals should be monitored for clinical signs of toxicity immediately after exposure, e.g. 1 min, 0.5 h, 1 h, 2 h and 4 h post-dosing. Daily observations may be sufficient where repeated treatments are used.

Consistent procedures for recording clinical signs and determining compound toxicity should be adopted during the toxicity study and dominant lethal test to co-ordinate findings and trends.

It is recommended that a gross post-mortem examination is performed on unscheduled animal deaths to identify toxicity in potential target organs and possible causes of lethality.

6.4.6 Fertility testing

The fecundity of the rodent species and strain should ideally be known. If not, a pre-trial fertility study may prove informative, especially when a test agent is suspected of affecting the sexual behaviour of the animal, e.g. due to changes in hormonal or physiological status (Ray & Hyneck, 1973).

A net decrease in the numbers of litters observed may be the result of either a reduced mating frequency and/or a reduced fertilisation rate of the eggs. The former situation is usually associated with compound toxicity while the latter may have genotoxic causes.

To determine the actual level of pre-implantation losses accurately in the dominant lethal assay, it is necessary to confirm both that matings have occurred (Section 6.4.2) and to examine cytologically the number of fertilised ova in the exposed animals (Kratochvilova, 1978). However, for practical purposes the latter analysis is usually omitted from routine testing.

At the end of the dominant lethal test, supplementary assays may be undertaken on partly or completely sterile males to investigate potential damage to their reproductive tracts. Such assessments may include testicular and epididymal weight, as well as sperm density and abnormality (Conner *et al.*, 1990). Gross deviations in any of these measurements are usually associated with a reduction in fertility, although inherited cytogenetic defects may also be responsible (Morissey *et al.*, 1988; Generoso *et al.*, 1990).

Histopathological examination of abnormal testes should be carried out if an increased number of treated animals. e.g. > 10%, within any one dose group, shows a marked impairment of fertilising capacity during the dominant lethal assay. Such an approach may help to confirm germ cell damage in the case of a weak dominant lethal effect (Murota, Shibuya & Iwahara, 1981; Saito-Suzuki *et al.*, 1982; Lane *et al.*, 1985).

6.5   ASSESSMENT DETAILS
6.5.1   Mating period

Mating schedules and frequencies have been described (Sections 6.2.1 and 6.4.2).

6.5.2   Assessment point

Mated females should be assessed at a pre-determined time in the later stages of pregnancy. For confirmed matings, this assessment is usually performed around 15 or 16 days post coitus in both mice and rats. In the absence of mating confirmation, it is common to assess animals 17 days from the first caging day. This assumes that most successful matings occur around the midpoint of the mating period so that the majority of embryos will be 13.5 days old at assessment, whenever the typical 7 or 4 day mating intervals are used.

Assessment, therefore, takes place when the embryo has reached the final stages of embryogenesis when organ formation is near completion. In rats and mice, organogenesis spans days 6–15 of embryonal life with a peak of activity around days 10–11. Parturition occurs 18–19 days after fertilisation in mice and 21–22 days after fertilisation in rats.

6.5.3.   Embryo observations

The primary indicators of a dominant lethal effect are:
1. a reduced number of live implants per female
2. a reduced number of total implants per female
3. a reduced number of pregnant females

These dominant lethal indicators have been described in detail by Epstein *et al.* (1970); Lyon & Smith (1971); Generoso *et al.* (1974); Singh, Lawrence & Autian (1974) and Moreland *et al* (1979).

A reduction in the numbers of implants can arise from both genotoxic and non-genotoxic causes operating at different points during the progression from mating to examination. When not due to a reduced mating frequency, the chief causes of such reductions are:
1. an increased number of pre-implantation losses (corpora lutea minus total implants)
2. an increased number of post-implantation losses (total implants minus live implants)
3. an increased number of pre-implantation and post-implantation losses (corpora lutea minus live implants)

6.5.3.1   Corpora lutea

The primary function of the corpus luteum (yellow body) is to secrete progesterone hormone which is required for the growth of the implanted egg. If, for whatever reason, the development of the egg is stopped, the corpus luteum will continue to grow for a period of time in the absence of an embryo. The number of corpora lutea is therefore an estimate of the total number of possible fertilisation events. When a significant decrease in the number of corpora lutea is observed, the following factors could be responsible: 1) a reduction in the number of ovulations; 2) a reduction in the number of fertilisations; 3) loss of corpora lutea due to embryo death.

It should be noted that counting corpora lutea accurately is difficult even when using a dissection microscope. Corpora lutea estimates in mice are frequently omitted for this reason (Ehling *et al.*, 1978).

6.5.3.2 Total implants

In dominant lethal testing, a reduction in litter size is indicative of reduced fertility in the exposed animals. Evident reductions in fertility or complete animal sterility is often linked to extensive spermatogonial cell damage and lack of sperm production (Searle & Beechey, 1974; Meistrich, 1982; Bucci & Meistrich, 1987). When cellular damage is confined to the pre-meiotic phase, it will therefore not be detected as an increase in dominant lethality, but as a decrease in the number of litters (Röhrborn, 1970; Murota *et al.*, 1981; Generoso *et al.*, 1989*b*). The earliest induction of dominant lethals appears to occur when differentiating spermatogonia are exposed to germ cell genotoxins during their pre-meiotic DNA synthetic phase (Epstein *et al.*, 1970; Generoso, Preston & Brewin, 1975; Ehling, 1977; Pandey *et al.*, 1990).

6.5.3.3 Live implants

The most critical aspect of dominant lethal assessment is to identify correctly the number of dead and live implants in each dose group. A live implant is a normally developed embryo which is in an advanced or completed state of organogenesis. Live embryos have a prominent, functioning blood vasculature with recognisable internal and external organs. They usually show movements within the amniotic sac.

6.5.3.4 Dead implants

A dead implant may show varying degrees of degeneration or necrosis. It is classified as being either an early or late death. An early death generally occurs before organogenesis begins, while a late death takes place in the immediate days before assessment when the organ formation is nearly complete.

Early deaths are recovered in the form of deciduomata or implantation 'moles'. The moles form part of the deciduum which is a growth of maternal uterine tissue in response to the stimuli emitted by the embryo. Early deaths frequently have a black appearance due to the presence of oxygenated and clotted blood around and within the partially resorbed embryo (Bateman, 1977; Anderson *et al.*, 1983).

Individual moles may vary considerably in size within and between animals.

In mice, physical dislocation of moles is common and careful dissection of the uterine horns is needed.

Several methods have been developed for the unambiguous verification of implantation traces left by early embryonal deaths or abortions. These include staining with dilute ammonium sulphide or, alternatively, ammonium hydroxide followed by formalin fixation for permanently stained preparations (Yamada *et al.*, 1985). Such relatively time-consuming techniques should only be used to clarify ambiguous dominant lethal effects.

Late embryo deaths are usually related to adverse environmental influences, e.g. microbial infections (Röhrborn, 1968). However, certain agents may also increase the frequency of such deaths (Singh *et al.*, 1974; Favor *et al.*, 1978). Late deaths are easily recognised by their distinct pale colour and the absence of a functioning blood vasculature. Puncture of the amniotic sac typically reveals an autolysed embryo.

6.6   DATA EVALUATION
6.6.1   Data presentation
Data from dominant lethal tests can be presented and analysed in a variety of ways. Some commonly examined variables in dominant lethal testing are shown in Table 6.2.

6.6.2   Statistical analysis
The treated animal is the unit of statistical analysis in any dominant lethal assay (Smith & James, 1984; Chanter *et al.*, 1989). The original methods used to analyse such data have been described (Anderson *et al.*, 1983). More recently, various procedures for evaluating dominating lethal data have been reviewed by Chanter *et al.* (1989) and Lockhart, Piegorsch & Bishop (1992). The range of statistical methods available reflects different approaches on how best to analyse the many variables measured and the complexity of the biological system studied.

Statistical methods which are simple to execute have advantages because computational and cumulative errors are minimised with respect to calculation, checking and presentation of the results. Expert statistical advice should be sought if there is any doubt on which method is appropriate for the analysis of a given observation.

For the analysis of direct proportions such as sterile males or fertilised females in different treatment groups, statistical approaches relying on chi-square methods, Fisher exact or permutation tests for comparison are generally sufficient (Green *et al.*, 1985; Chanter *et al.*, 1989).

Data for both pre-implantation and post-implantation losses often require more complex statistical treatment. Both non-parametric and parametric

Table 6.2.

Level	Variable examined
Ia	Number of females mated
b	Number of females plugged (vaginal plug/sperm positive)
c	Number of females pregnant
IIa	Number of corpora lutea per female
IIIa	Number of implantations per female
b	Number of pre-implantation losses per female (IIa–IIIa)
IVa	Number of live embryos per female
b	Number of dead embryos per female
Va	Number of early deaths per female
b	Number of late deaths per female
VIa	Proportion of females with one or more early deaths
b	Proportion of females with two or more early deaths
c	Proportion of females with two or less early deaths
d	Proportion of females with three or more early deaths

Table adapted from Ehling *et al.* (1978).

approaches can be used for analysis. The latter subdivide into those based on normal distribution or binomial distribution. If a parametric approach is chosen, it is normal to transform the data sets before analysis. Some commonly used means of transforming data and performing the subsequent statistical analyses, including discussions of interpretations, have been reviewed by Smith and James (1984), Chanter *et al.* (1989) and Lockhart *et al.* (1992).

Biological interpretation should be applied to statistical findings before drawing conclusions on dominant lethal effects. The critical issue is to achieve the correct balance between an understanding of reproductive biology and of statistical principles. Statistical decision rules should not be used in place of sound scientific judgements when evaluating experimental data (Haseman, 1990).

6.6.3 Biological interpretation

Appreciable group variations in post-implantation losses are often observed. In general, it is unusual for an individual control animal to show more than two early deaths per pregnancy (Epstein *et al.*, 1972; Haseman & Soares, 1976; Arnold *et al.*, 1976). Occasionally, however, individual females may show a high rate of death. Such findings may have a treatment-related basis and should be interpreted with caution (Roberts & Rand, 1978; Lane *et al.*, 1985).

In dominant lethal tests using treated males, acute or subacute agent exposures allow for a general separation of germ cell damage into pre-meiotic,

meiotic and post-meiotic effects. During chronic dosing, no such distinction is possible as all germ cell stages have been exposed repeatedly. In male mice and rats, post-meiotic sperm effects induced by acute or subacute treatments will be readily detected during the first 3 weeks of mating. Later matings will represent a mixture of meiotically and pre-meiotically exposed sperm. For this reason, it may be justified to pool data across relevant weeks in order to evaluate trends over the major spermatogenic stages (Green & Springer, 1973; Green *et al.*, 1985).

6.6.4   Negative findings

A negative dominant lethal response is presumed if neither pre-implantation nor post-implantation losses can be demonstrated in the various treatment groups under the defined statistical and/or biological criteria of the assay. Statistically significant increases at the 5% level over relevant control points are usually considered indicative of a dominant lethal effect (see Section 6.5.3). However, as it is not unusual to obtain sporadic significances at the 5% level in individual assessment weeks, it is essential that the statistical findings are considered in a historical context with regard to spontaneous levels of dominant lethal induction and normal biological variability (Green & Springer, 1973; Arnold *et al.*, 1976; Lane *et al.*, 1985). In certain cases, it may be desirable to support the negative findings with metabolic and pharmacokinetic data to confirm that a compound reaches the germ cells (Dixon & Lee, 1973; Setchell, 1980) without inducing dominant lethal effects following a given regimen (Khera *et al.*, 1976; Simon *et al.*, 1986).

6.6.5   Positive findings

A positive dominant lethal effect is presumed if any one of the indicators described in Section 6.5.3 shows a statistically significant and biologically meaningful difference from the negative control group. More often than not, a true dominant lethal effect will be demonstrated by differences in more than one of the three primary criteria. Dominant lethal effects are usually dose-dependent and occur in more than one assessment (Green & Springer, 1973; Arnold *et al.*, 1976; Moreland *et al.*, 1979). Male sterility during the most sensitive gametogenic stage is also often observed (Generoso *et al.*, 1974; Searle & Beechey, 1974; McGregor *et al.*, 1983).

6.6.6   Ambiguous findings

Several chemicals which have been reported in the literature to have given positive results in the dominant lethal assay have on retesting, using more rigorous protocols and/or techniques, failed to induce positive responses. These discrepancies may be due to a variety of causes, such as poor study design, application of unsuitable statistical methods and the failure to interpret the results in a biological context. Caution is therefore advised when evaluating any borderline or weak dominant lethal effects (Simon, Tardiff & Borzelleca, 1978; Lane *et al.*, 1985). It is recommended that particular attention is given to concurrent vehicle control effects across the assessment period, as well as to any relevant historical data base (Epstein *et al.*, 1972). If the issue cannot be resolved via such approaches, the assay should be repeated. Unexplained variations in dominant lethal responses should be carefully checked against the laboratory environmental records for the study (Röhrborn, 1968; Garriott and Chrisman, 1981).

6.6.7 Dose responses

A common observation in dominant lethal testing is that of different dominant lethal effects at different doses of compound. Thus, whereas a low dose may only target a particular stage of spermatogenesis, higher agent doses will affect a greater number of meiotic stages (Generoso *et al.*, 1975; Schreiner & Steelman, 1977; Ehling & Neuhäuser-Klaus, 1989).

Dose–responses in dominant lethal induction may vary significantly. Thus, triethylenemelamine induces dominant lethality in exposed males in a linear, dose-related fashion (Matter & Generoso, 1974). Other genotoxins such as ethyl methanesulphonate and ethylene oxide show a much steeper, non-linear dose–response (Generoso *et al.*, 1974; Rhomberg *et al.*, 1990). Inconsistent or atypical dose–responses, e.g. because only some females show an effect at a given dose, may also occur (Roberts & Rand, 1978; Moreland *et al.*, 1979; Badr, Rabouh & Badr, 1979). Dose–responses in the dominant lethal test have been discussed by Epstein *et al.* (1970), Generoso *et al.* (1974) and Arnold *et al.* (1976).

Toxic interferences with gamete production and maturation should be suspected where greater or comparable induction of dominant lethals occurs at low relative to high compound doses (Simon *et al.*, 1978).

6.6.8 Repeat studies

Dominant lethal tests which give rise to inconclusive results as determined by statistical and/or biological criteria should be repeated if necessary, but with careful justification in view of the numbers of animals used. In any repeat assay, particular attention must be given to 1) the nature of the initial response; 2) the dose at which the effect occurred; 3) the particular gametogenic stage showing an increase in dominant lethals; 4) the metabolic and pharmacokinetic behaviour of the compound and its main metabolites; 5) the possibility of a sex-dependent effect in dominant lethal induction; 6) the suitability of the dominant lethal test to assess the obtained effect.

6.7   CONCLUSIONS

The primary role of the dominant lethal assay is to evaluate genotoxic effects on germ cells following positive test results from *in vivo* somatic assays. A positive dominant lethal test provides a quantifiable measure of damage to the germ cells, especially when males are treated. Dominant lethality is frequently caused by cytogenetic damage although other genetic or epigenetic lesions may also be involved.

Positive results from the dominant lethal assay may help to predict which spermatogenic stages are likely to show responses in other germ cell assays (Nagao, 1988; Russell *et al.*, 1989; Ehling & Neuhäuser-Klaus, 1989). However, negative dominant lethal findings do not exclude the possibility of underlying genetic damage in the exposed germ cells (Adler & El Tarras, 1990). The absence of embryonic death can therefore not be equated with the absence of germ cell damage, given the relative resilience of the spermatogenic process and the use of females to assess for effects on males. The dominant lethal test also does not supply information on heritable hazard because the specific endpoint assessed is embryo death.

In dominant lethal testing, treatment of males is far more common as it largely eliminates the problem of separating toxic and genotoxic effects within the organism. The rodent dominant lethal test can be performed using acute, subacute or chronic dosing regimens. Common dose routes of administration are oral and intraperitoneal exposures, although other routes can also be used.

The rodent dominant lethal test is a relatively time-consuming and expensive short-term animal assay for genotoxicity. It is, therefore, especially important that the biological principles and limitations are understood before an experiment is performed. Factors requiring special attention include: 1) the expected size and stage-specificity of the dominant lethal effect; 2) the normal biological variability of the test system using the study design in question; 3) the economics and ethics of testing as regards animal numbers and experimental regimen; 4) the choice of the statistical methods used to analyse for dominant lethality.

These complex and interacting concerns frequently necessitate a flexible approach to testing and an acceptable compromise between scientific and practical concerns. The study design adopted should, however, always reflect the pre-set objectives of the assay and the actual observations to be made during the dominant lethal experiment.

Where the dominant lethal test is used in its recommended role, as a germ cell assay for the evaluation of compounds with known genotoxic potential in somatic cells *in vivo*, the following routine testing strategy is suitable. A minimum of 15 males are treated via the chosen dose route for 2–5 days, typically using three dose levels in which the highest dose induces a measure of toxicity, before successive mating of the exposed males to virgin females using 1:1, 1:2 or 1:3 caging ratios and the preferred mating interval.

Where a female dominant lethal assay is conducted, due to a suspected sex difference in responsiveness, the same dosing and mating objectives apply as for the male assay. Positive findings in the female dominant lethal test should be analysed further via cytogenetic and/or other methods to confirm the genetic nature of the obtained response.

6.8 REFERENCES

Adler, I-D. & Brewen, J. G. (1982). Effects of chemicals on chromosome aberration production in male and female germ cells. In *Chemical Mutagens. Principles and Methods for their Detection*, eds. A. Hollaender and F. J. de Serres, vol. 7, Plenum Press, New York, pp. 1–35.

Adler, I-D. & El Tarras, A. (1990). Clastogenic effects of cisdiamminedichloroplatinum II. Induction of chromosomal aberrations in primary spermatocytes and spermatogonial stem cells of mice. *Mutation Research*, **243**, 173–8.

Amann, P. (1989). Structure and function of the normal testis and epididymis. *Journal of the American College of Toxicology*, **8**, 457–71.

Anderson, D., Bateman, A. & McGregor, D. (1983). Dominant lethal mutation assays. In *UKEMS Sub-committee on Guidelines for Mutagenicity Testing*. United Kingdom Environmental Mutagen Society, Swansea, pp. 143–64.

Anderson, D., Brinkworth, M. H., Jenkinson, P. C., Clode, S. A., Creasy, D. M. & Gangolli, S. D. (1987). Effect of ethylene glycol monomethyl ether on spermatogenesis, dominant lethality, and F_1 abnormalities in the rat and the mouse after treatment of F_0 males. *Teratogenesis, Carcinogenesis and Mutagenesis*, **7**, 141–58.

Arni, P., Ashby, S., Castellino, S., Engelhardt, G., Herbold, B. A., Priston, R. A. J. & Bontinck, W. J. (1988). Assessment of the potential germ cell mutagenicity of industrial and plant protection chemicals as part of an integrated study of genotoxicity *in vitro* and *in vivo*. *Mutation Research*, **203**, 177–84.

Arnold, D. W., Kennedy, G. L. Jr., Keplinger, M. L. & Calandra, J. C. (1976). Dominant lethal studies with alkylating agents: dose–response relationships. *Toxicology and Applied Pharmacology*, **38**, 79–84.

Ashby, J. (1986). The prospects for a simplified and internationally harmonized approach to the detection of possible human carcinogens and mutagens. *Mutagenesis*, **1**, 3–16.

Ashby, J. (1987). The efficient preparation of corn oil suspensions. *Mutation Research*, **187**, 45.

Au, W. W., Cantelli-Forti, G., Hrelia, P. & Legator, M. S. (1990). Cytogenetic assays in genotoxic studies: somatic cell effects of benzene and germinal cell effects of dibromochloropropane. *Teratogenesis, Carcinogenesis and Mutagenesis*, **10**, 125–34.

Badr, F. M. & Badr, R. S. (1974). Studies on the mutagenic effects of contraceptive drugs. I. Induction of dominant lethal mutations in female mice. *Mutation Research*, **26**, 529–34.

Badr, F. M., Rabouh, S. A. & Badr, R. S. (1979). On the mutagenicity of methadone hydrochloride. Induced dominant lethal mutation and spermatocyte chromosomal aberrations in treated males. *Mutation Research*, **68**, 235–49.

Bateman, A. J. (1958). The partition of dominant lethals in the mouse between unimplanted eggs and deciduomata. *Heredity*, **12**, 467–75.

Bateman, A. J. (1977). The dominant lethal assay in the male mouse. In *Handbook of Mutagenicity Test Procedures*, eds. B. Kilbey, M. Legator, W. Nichols and C. Ramel, Elsevier, Amsterdam, pp. 325–34.

Bishop, J. B., Kodell, R. L., Whorton, E. B. & Domon, O. E. (1983). Dominant lethal test response with IMS and TEM using different combinations of male and female stocks of mice. *Mutation Research*, **121**, 273–80.

Brandriff, R. & Pedersen, R. A. (1981). Repair of the ultraviolet-irradiated male genome in fertilised mouse eggs. *Science*, **211**, 1431.

Brewen, J. G. & Payne, H. S. (1976). Studies on chemically induced dominant lethality. II. Cytogenetic study of MMS-induced dominant lethality in maturing dictyate mouse oocytes. *Mutation Research*, **37**, 77–82.

Bucci, L. R. & Meistrich, M. L. (1987). Effects of busulfan on murine spermatogenesis: cytotoxicity, sterility, sperm abnormalities, and dominant lethal mutations. *Mutation Research*, **176**, 259–68.

Chanter, D. O., Anderson, D., Bateman, A., Lovell, D. P., Palmer, A. K., Stevens, M. T. & Richold, M. (1989). Statistical methods for the dominant lethal assay. In *UKEMS Sub-Committee on Guidelines for Mutagenicity Testing. Report. Part III. Statistical Evaluation of Mutagenicity Test Data*, ed. D. J. Kirkland, Cambridge University Press, Cambridge, pp. 233–50.

Chellman, G. J., Bus, J. S. G. & Working, P. K. (1986). Role of epididymal inflammation in the induction of dominant lethal mutations in Fischer 344 rat sperm by methyl chloride. *Proceedings of the National Academy of Sciences, USA*, **83**, 8087–91.

Clermont, Y. (1972). Kinetics of spermatogenesis in mammals: seminiferous epithelium cycle and spermatogenical renewal. *Physiological Reviews*, **52**, 198–236.

Conner, M. W., Conner, B. H., Rogers, A. E. & Newberne, P. M. (1990). Anguidine-induced testicular injury in Lewis rats. *Reproductive Toxicology*, **4**, 215–22.

Dean, B. J. & Johnstone, A. (1977). Dominant lethal assays in male mice: evaluation of experimental design, statistical methods and the sensitivity of Charles River (CD1) mice. *Mutation Research*, **42**, 269–78.

Dean, B. J., Anderson, D. & Srám, R. J. (1981). Mutagenicity of selected chemicals in the mammalian dominant lethal assay. In *Comparative Chemical Mutagenesis*, eds. F. J. de Serres and M. D. Shelby, Plenum Press, pp. 487–538.

De Pass, L. R. (1989). Alternative approaches in median lethality (LD_{50}) and acute toxicity testing. *Toxicology Letters*, **49**, 159–70.

DH (1989). Guidelines for the testing of chemicals for mutagenicity. *Department of Health Report on Health and Social Subjects* No. 35. HMSO, London.

Dixon, R. L. & Lee, I. P. (1973). Possible role of the blood–testicular barrier in dominant lethal testing. *Environmental Health Perspectives*, **6**, 59–66.

EEC (in press). Methods for the determination of physico-chemical properties, toxicity and ecotoxicity: *Annex V to Directive 67/548/EEC*. Tests B1, B2, B3 and B12 (revisions in progress).

Ehling, U. H. (1977). Dominant lethal mutations in male mice. *Archives of Toxicology*, **38**, 1–11.

Ehling, U. H., Machemer, L., Buselmaier, W., Dycka, J., Frohberg, H., Kratochvilova, J., Lang, R., Lorke, D., Müller, D., Peh, J., Röhrborn, G., Roll, R., Schulze-Schencking, M. & Wiemann, H. (1978). Standard protocol for the dominant lethal test on male mice. Set up by the work group 'Dominant Lethal Mutations of the *ad hoc* Committee Chemogenetics', *Archives of Toxicology*, **39**, 173–85.

Ehling, U. H. & Neuhäuser-Klaus, A. (1989). Induction of specific-locus and dominant lethal mutations in male mice by chloromethine. *Mutation Research*, **227**, 81–9.

Ehling, U. H. & Neuhäuser-Klaus, A. (1990). Induction of specific-locus and dominant lethal mutations in male mice in the low dose range by methyl methanesulphonate (MMS). *Mutation Research*, **230**, 61–70.

Epstein, S. S. & Shafner, H. (1968). Chemical mutagens in the human environment. *Nature*, **219**, 385–7.

Epstein, S. S., Arnold, E., Steinberg, K., Mackintosh, D., Shafner, H. & Bishop, Y. (1970). Mutagenic and antifertility effects of TEPA and METEPA in mice. *Toxicology and Applied Pharmacology*, **17**, 23–40.

Epstein, S. S., Arnold, E., Andrea, J., Bass, W. & Bishop, Y. (1972). Detection of chemical mutagens by the dominant lethal assay in the mouse. *Toxicology and Applied Pharmacology*, **23**, 288–325.

Erickson, P. (1990). Post-meiotic gene expression. *Trends in Genetics*, **6**, 264–9.

Favor, J., Soares, E. R. & Crenshaw, J. W., Jr. (1978). Chemical and radiation induced late dominant lethal effects in mice. *Mutation Research*, **54**, 333–42.

Favor, J. (1990). Multiple endpoint mutational analysis in the mouse. *Progress in Clinical and Biological Research*, **340C**, 115–24.

Fielder, R. J., Allen, J. A., Boobis, A. R., Botham, P. A., Doe, J., Esdaile, D. J., Gatehouse, D. G., Hodson-Walker, G., Morton, D. B., Kirkland, D. J. & Richold, M. (1992). Report of British Toxicology Society/UK Environmental Mutagen Society Working Group. Dose Setting in *in vivo* Mutagenicity Assays. *Mutagenesis*, **7**, 313–19.

Fox, B. W. & Fox, M. (1967). Biochemical aspects of the action of drugs on spermatogenesis. *Pharmacological Reviews*, **19**, 21–57.

Garriott, M. L. & Chrisman, C. L. (1981). Investigation of hyperthermia-induced dominant lethal mutations in male mice. *The Journal of Heredity*, **72**, 338–42.

Generoso, W. M., Russell, W. L., Huff, S. W., Stout, S. K. & Gosslee, D. G. (1974). Effects of dose on the induction of dominant-lethal mutations and heritable translocations with ethyl methanesulfonate in male mice. *Genetics*, **77**, 741–52.

Generoso, W. M., Preston, R. J. & Brewen, J. C. (1975). 6-mercaptopurine, an inducer of cytogenetic and dominant lethal effects in premeiotic and early meiotic germ cells of male mice. *Mutation Research*, **28**, 437–47.

Generoso, W. M., Cumming, R. B., Bandy, J. A. & Cain, K. T. (1983). Increased dominant-lethal effects due to prolonged exposure of mice to inhaled ethylene oxide. *Mutation Research*, **119**, 377–9.

Generoso, W. M., Cain, K. T., Hoskins, J. A., Washington, W. J. & Rutledge, J. C. (1984). Pseudo dominant-lethal response in female mice treated with plant oils. *Mutation Research*, **129**, 235–41.

Generoso, W. M., Cain, K. T. & Hughes, L. A. (1985). Tests for dominant lethal effects of 1,2-dibromo-3-chloro-propane (DBCP) in male and female mice. *Mutation Research*, **156**, 103–8.

Generoso, W. M., Katoh, M., Cain, K. T., Hughes, L. A., Foxworth, L. B., Mitchell, T. J. & Bishop, J. A. (1989*a*). Chromosome malsegregation and embryonic lethality induced by treatment of normally ovulated mouse oocytes with nocodazole. *Mutation Research*, **210**, 313–22.

Generoso, W. M., Cain, K. T., Hughes, L. A. & Foxworth, L. B. (1989*b*). A restudy of the efficacy of adriamycin in inducing dominant lethals in mouse spermatogonial stem cells. *Mutation Resarch*, **226**, 61–4.

Generoso, W. M., Cain, K. T., Cornett, C. V., Cachiero, N. L. A. and Hughes, L. A. (1990). Concentration–response curves for ethylene-oxide-induced heritable translocations and dominant lethal mutations. *Environmental and Molecular Mutagenesis*, **16**, 126–31.

Grahn, D., Carnes, B. A. & Farrington, B. H. (1986). Genetic injury in hybrid male mice exposed to low doses of ^{60}Co gamma-rays or fission neutrons. II. Dominant lethal mutation response to long-term weekly exposures. *Mutation Research*, **162**, 81–9.

Green, S. & Springer, J. A. (1973). The dominant-lethal test: potential limitations and statistical considerations for safety evaluation. *Environmental Health Perspectives*, **6**, 37–46.

Green, S., Carr, J. V., Sauro, F. M. & Legator, M. S. (1973). Effects of hycanthone on spermatogonical cells, deoxyribonucleic acid synthesis in bone marrow and dominant lethality in rats. *Journal of Pharmacology and Experimental Therapy*, **187**, 437–43.

Green, S., Auletta, A., Fabricant, J., Kapp, R., Manandhar, M., Sheu, C.-J., Springer, J. & Whitfield, B. (1985). Current status of bioassays in genetic toxicology – the dominant lethal assay. A Report of the US Environmental Protection Agency Gene-Tox Program. *Mutation Research*, **154**, 49–67.

Hardin, B. D. (1983). Reproductive toxicity of the glycol ethers. *Toxicology*, **27**, 91–102.

Hansmann, I. (1974). Chromosome aberrations in metaphase II-oocytes. Stage sensitivity in the mouse oogenesis to amethopterin and cyclophosphamide. *Mutation Research*, **22**, 175–91.

Haseman, J. K. & Soares, E. R. (1976). The distribution of fetal death in control mice and its implications on statistical tests for dominant lethal effects. *Mutation Research*, **41**, 277–88.

Haseman, J. K. (1990). Use of statistical decision rules for evaluating laboratory animal carcinogenicity studies. *Fundamental and Applied Toxicology*, **14**, 637–48.

Hess, R. (1973). Induced dominant lethals in female mice. *Agents and Actions*, **3**, 116–17.

Hitotsumachi, S. & Kikuchi, Y. (1977). Chromosome aberrations and dominant lethality of mouse embryos after paternal treatment with triethylenemelamine. *Mutation Research*, **42**, 117–24.

HMSO (1990). Her Majesty's Stationery Office. *Guidance on the Operation of Animals (Scientific Procedures) Act 1986*. Publication No. 182, HMSO, London.

Holden, H. E. (1982). Comparison of somatic and germ cell models for cytogenetic screening. *Journal of Applied Toxicology*, **2**, 196–200.

Holliday, R. (1987). The inheritance of epigenetic defects. *Science*, **238**, 163–70.

Katoh, M. A., Cain, K. T., Hughes, L. A., Foxworth, L. B., Bishop, J. B. & Generoso, W. M. (1990). Female-specific dominant lethal effects in mice. *Mutation Research*, **230**, 205–17.

Khera, K. S., Villeneuve, D. C., Terry, G., Panopio, L., Nash, L. & Trivett, G. (1976). Mirex: a teratogenicity, dominant lethal and tissue distribution study in rats. *Food and Chemical Toxicology*, **14**, 25–9.

Kratochvilova, J. (1978). Evaluation of pre-implantation loss in dominant-lethal assay in the mouse. *Mutation Research*, **54**, 47–54.

Kuhlmann, W. (1970). Cytology and timing of meiotic stages in female germ cells of mammals and man. In *Chemical Mutagenesis in Mammals and Man*, eds. F. Vogel and G. Röhrborn, Springer, Berlin, pp. 180–93.

Lane, R. W., Simon, G. S., Dougherty, R. W., Egle, J. L., Jr. & Borzelleca, J. F. (1985). Reproductive toxicity and lack of dominant lethal effects of 2,4-dinitrotoluene in the male rat. *Drug and Chemical Toxicology*, **8**, 265–80.

Leblond, C. P. & Clermont, Y. (1952). Spermiogenesis of rat, mouse, hamster and guinea pig as revealed by the 'periodic acid-fuchsin sulphurous' technique. *American Journal of Anatomy*, **90**, 167–216.

Lee, I. P. (1983). Adaptive biochemical repair response toward germ cell DNA damage. *American Journal of Industrial Medicine*, **4**, 135–47.

Lee, K. P. & Kinney, L. A. (1989). The ultrastructure and reversibility of testicular atrophy induced by ethylene glycol monomethyl ether (EGME) in the rat. *Toxicologic Pathology*, **17**, 759–73.

Léonard, A., Deknudt, G., Linden, G. & Gilliavod, N. (1972). Strain variations in the incidence of dominant lethals induced by X-irradiation given to mouse spermatozoa. *Strahlentherapie*, **143**, 102–5.

Lockhart, A.-M. C., Piegorsch, W. W. & Bishop, J. B. (1992). Assessing overdispersion and dose–response in the male dominant lethal assay. *Mutation Research*, **272**, 35–58.

Lovell, D. P., Anderson, D. & Jenkinson, P. C. (1987). The use of a battery of mice in a factorial design to study the induction of dominant lethal mutation. *Mutation Research*, **187**, 37–44.

Lyon, M. F. & Smith, B. D. (1971). Species comparisons concerning radiation-induced dominant lethals and chromosome aberrations. *Mutation Research*, **11**, 45–58.

Lyon, M. F. (1981). Sensitivity of various germ-cell stages to environmental mutagens. ICPEMC Working Paper 4/1. *Mutation Research*, **87**, 323–45.

Mackay, J. M. & Elliott, B. M. (1992). Dose-ranging and dose-setting for *in vivo* genetic toxicology studies. *Mutation Research*, **271**, 97–9.

Mailhes, J. B., Yuan, Z. P. & Aardema, M. J. (1990). Cytogenetic analysis of mouse oocytes and one-cell zygotes as a potential assay for heritable germ cell aneuploidy. *Mutation Research*, **242**, 89–100.

Mailhes, J. B. & Aardema, M. J. (1992). Benomyl-induced aneuploidy in mouse oocytes. *Mutagenesis*, **7**, 303–9.

Matter, B. E. & Generoso, W. M. (1974). Effect of dose on the induction of dominant lethal mutations with triethylenemelamine in male mice. *Genetics*, **77**, 753–63.

Matter, B. E. & Jaeger, I. (1975). Premature chromosome condensation, structural chromosome aberrations and micronuclei in early mouse embryos after treatment of paternal post-meiotic germ cells with triethylenemelamine, possible mechanisms for chemically induced dominant-lethal mutations. *Mutation Research*, **33**, 251–60.

Mattison, D. R. & Thomford, P. J. (1989). The mechanisms of action of reproductive toxicants. *Toxicologic Pathology*, **17**, 364–76.

Maxwell, W. A. & Newell, G. W. (1973). Considerations for evaluating chemical mutagenicity to germinal cells. *Environmental Health Perspectives*, **6**, 47–50.

McGregor, D. B., Willins, M. J., McDonald, P., Holmstrom, M., McDonald, D. & Niemeier, R. W. (1983). Genetic effects of 2-methoxyethanol and bis(2-methoxyethyl)ether. *Toxicology and Applied Pharmacology*, **70**, 303–16.

Meistrich, M. L. (1982). Quantitative correlation between testicular stem cell survival, sperm production, and fertility in the mouse after treatment with different cytotoxic agents. *Journal of Andrology*, **3**, 58–68.

Meistrich, M. L. (1986). Critical components of testicular function and sensitivity to disruption. *Biology of Reproduction*, **34**, 17–28.

Moreland, F. M., Kilian, D. J., Palmer, A. K., Springer, J. A., Green, S. & Legator, M. (1979). A collaborative dominant lethal study of triethylenemelamine in the rat. *Toxicology and Applied Pharmacology*, **49**, 161–70.

Morissey, R. E., Lamb *IV*, J. C., Schwetz, B. A., Teague, J. L. & Morris, R. W. (1988). Association of sperm, vaginal cytology and reproductive organ weight data with results of continuous breeding reproduction studies in Swiss (CD-1) mice. *Toxicology and Applied Pharmacology*, **11**, 359–71.

Murota, T., Shibuya, T. & Iwahara, S. (1981). Dominant lethal testing of 7,12-dimethylbenz(α)anthracene with spermatogenic cells of mice. *Mutation Research*, **91**, 273–7.

Nagao, T. (1988). Congenital defects in the offspring of male mice treated with ethylnitrosourea. *Mutation Research*, **202**, 25–33.

Oakberg, E. F. (1956). Duration of spermatogenesis in the mouse and timing of stages of the cycle of the seminiferous epithelium. *American Journal of Anatomy*, **99**, 507–16.

Oakberg, E. F. (1979). Timing of oocyte maturation in the mouse and its relevance to radiation-induced cell killing and mutational sensitivity. *Mutation Research*, **59**, 39–48.

Pandey, H., Gundevia, F., Prem, A. S. & Ray, P. K. (1990). Studies on the genotoxicity of endosulfan, an organochlorine insecticide, in mammalian germ cells. *Mutation Research*, **242**, 1–7.

Paolini, M., Biagi, G. L. & Forti, G. C. (1988). The efficient preparation of corn oil solutions. *Mutation Research*, **206**, 127–8.

Pathki, V. & Polasa, H. (1988). Dominant lethality in mice – a test for mutagenicity of influenza X-31 virus. *Teratogenesis, Carcinogenesis and Mutagenesis*, **8**, 55–62.

Propping, P., Röhrborn, G. & Buselmaier, W. (1972). Comparative investigations on the chemical induction of point mutations and dominant lethal mutations in mice. *Molecular and General Genetics*, **117**, 197–209.

Ray, V. A. & Hyneck, M. L. (1973). Some primary considerations in the interpretation of the dominant-lethal assay. *Environmental Health Perspectives*, **6**, 27–35.

Reddi, O. S. & Vasudevan, B. (1968). Induced dominant lethality in mice by phosphorus-32. *Nature*, **218**, 283–4.

Rhomberg, L., Dellarco, V. L., Siegel-Scott, C., Dearfield, K. L. & Jacobson-Kram, D. (1990). Quantitative estimation of the genetic risks associated with the induction of heritable translocations at low-dose exposure. Ethylene oxide as an example. *Environmental and Molecular Mutagenesis*, **16**, 104–25.

Roberts, G. T. & Rand, M. J. (1978). The dominant lethal effects of some ergot alkaloids. *Mutation Research*, **50**, 317–25.

Roberts, A., Renwick, A. G., Ford, G., Creasy, D. M. & Gaunt, I. (1989). The metabolism and toxicity of cychlohexylamine in rats and mice during chronic dietary administration. *Toxicology and Applied Pharmacology*, **98**, 216–29.

Röhrborn, G. (1968). Mutagenicity tests in mice. I. The dominant lethal method and the control problem. *Humangenetik*, **6**, 345–51.

Röhrborn, G. (1970). The activity of alkylating agents. I. Sensitive mutable stages in spermatogenesis and oogenesis. In *Chemical Mutagenesis in Mammals and Man*, eds. F. Vogel and G. Röhrborn, Springer, Berlin, pp. 294–316.

Röhrborn, G. & Hansmann, I. (1974). Oral contraceptives and chromosome segregation in oocytes of mice. *Mutation Research*, **26**, 535–44.

Russell, L. B. & Shelby, M. D. (1985). Tests for heritable genetic damage and for evidence of gonadal exposure in mammals. *Mutation Research*, **154**, 69–84.

Russell, L. B., Hunsicker, P. R., Cacheiro, N. L. A., Bangham, J. W., Russell, W. L. & Shelby, M. D. (1989). Chlorambucil effectively induces deletion mutations in mouse germ cells. *Proceedings of the National Academy of Sciences, USA*, **86**, 3704–8.

Saito-Suzuki, R., Teramoto, S. & Shirasu, Y. (1982). Dominant lethal studies in rats with 1.2-dibromo-3-chloropropane and its structurally related compounds. *Mutation Research*, **101**, 321–7.

Schreiner, C. A. & Steelman, J. R. (1977). Oral triethylenemelamine: effects in the dominant lethal mutagenicity assay. *Toxicology and Applied Pharmacology*, **42**, 487–95.

Searle, A. G. & Beechey, C. V. (1974). Sperm count, egg-fertilization and dominant lethality after X-irradiation of mice. *Mutation Research*, **22**, 63–72.

Searle, A. G. & Beechey, C. V. (1985). The influence of mating status and age on the induction of chromosome aberrations and dominant lethals in irradiated female mice. *Mutation Research*, **147**, 357–62.

Setchell, B. P. (1980). The functional significance of the blood–testis barrier. *Journal of Andrology*, **1**, 3–10.

Shelby, M. D., Cain, K. T., Hughes, L. A., Braden, P. W. & Generoso, W. M. (1986). Dominant lethal effects of acrylamide in male mice. *Mutation Research*, **173**, 35–40.

Sheu, C.-J.W. & Moreland, F. M. (1983). Detection of dominant lethal mutation in mice after repeated low-dose administration of 6-mercaptopurine. *Drug and Chemical Toxicology*, **6**, 83–92.

Shibuya, T., Mijamae, Y. & Murota, T. (1988). Mouse dominant lethal test on four chemicals. In *International Programme on Chemical Safety. Evaluation of Short-term Tests for Carcinogens*, vol. 2, eds. J. Ashby, F. J. Serres, M. D. Shelby, B. H. Margolin, M. Ishidate Jr. and G. C. Becking, Cambridge University Press, Cambridge, pp. 208–14.

Simon, G. S., Tardiff, R. G. & Borzelleca, J. F. (1978). Potential mutagenic and adverse male reproductive effects of 1,2,3,4-tetrabromobutane: a dominant lethal study in the rat. *Toxicology and Applied Pharmacology*, **44**, 661–4.

Simon, G. S., Egle, J. L. Jr., Doughtery, R. W. & Borzelleca, J. F. (1986). Dominant lethal assay of chlordecone and its distribution in the male reproductive tissues of the rat. *Toxicology Letters*, **30**, 237–45.

Simula, A. P. & Priestly, B. G. (1991). Influence of vegetable oil vehicles on bone-marrow proliferation in the mouse micronucleus test. *Mutation Research*, **261**, 83–4.

Singh, A. R., Lawrence, W. H. & Autian, J. (1974). Mutagenic and anti-fertility sensitivities of mice to di(2-ethylhexyl)phthalate (DEPH) and dimethoxyethylphthalate (DMEP). *Toxicology and Applied Pharmacology*, **29**, 35–46.

Smith, D. M. & James, D. A. (1984). A comparison of alternative distributions of postimplantation death in the dominant lethal assay. *Mutation Research*, **128**, 195–206.

Soares, E. R. & Sheridan, W. (1977). Triethylenemelamine induced dominant lethals in mice – comparisons of oral versus intraperitoneal injection. *Mutation Research*, **43**, 247–54.

Sudman, P. D. & Generoso, W. M. (1991). Female-specific mutagenic response of mice to hycanthone. *Mutation Research*, **246**, 31–43.

Sẏkora, I. (1981). Dominant-lethal test of 6-mercaptopurine: dependence on dosage, duration and route of administration. *Neoplasma*, **28**, 739–46.

Tariq, M., Qureshi, S., Ageel, A. M. & Al-Meshal, I. A. (1990). The induction of dominant lethal mutations upon chronic administration of khat (Catha edulis) in albino mice. *Toxicology Letters*, **50**, 349–53.

Thompson, E. D. & Gibson, D. P. (1984). A method for determining the maximum tolerated dose for acute *in vivo* cytogenetic studies. *Food and Chemical Toxicology*, **22**, 665–76.

Trasler, J. M., Hales, B. F. & Robaire, B. (1986). Chronic low dose cyclophosphamide treatment of adult male rats: effect on fertility, pregnancy outcome and progeny. *Biology of Reproduction*, **34**, 275–83.

UFAW (1987). University Federation of Animal Welfare. *Handbook of Care and Management of Laboratory Animals*, ed. T. Poole. 6th edn, Longman Scientific and Technical, Essex, England.

Van den Heuvel, M. J., Clark, D. G., Fielder, R. J., Koundakjian, P. P., Oliver, G. J. A., Pelling, D., Tomlinson, N. J. & Walker, A. P. (1990). The international validation of a fixed dose procedure as an alternative to the classical LD_{50} test. *Food and Chemical Toxicology*, **28**, 469–82.

Verschaeve, L. & Léonard, A. (1984). Dominant lethality test in female mice treated with methyl mercury chloride. *Mutation Research*, **136**, 131–5.

Wallig, M. A., Gould, D. H., van Steenhouse, J., Fettman, M. J. & Willhite, C. C. (1989). The relationship of vehicle to target organ toxicology induced by the naturally occurring nitrile 1-cyano-2-hydroxy-3-butene. *Fundamental and Applied Toxicology*, **12**, 377–85.

Working, P. K., Bentley, K. S., Hurtt, M. E. & Mohr, K. L. (1987). Comparison of the dominant lethal effects of acrylonitrile and acrylamide in male Fischer 344 rats. *Mutagenesis*, **2**, 215–20.

Working, P. K. (1989). Mechanistic approaches in the study of testicular toxicology: agents that directly affect the testis. *Toxicologic Pathology*, **17**, 452–6.

Yamada, T., Hara, M., Ohba, Y., Inoue, T. & Ohno, H. (1985). Studies on implantation traces in rats. I. Size, observation period and staining. *Experimental Animals*, **34**, 17–22.

INDEX